Praise for
Resilient and Sustainable Caring

"Karen's timely work goes beyond the resiliency support we see in health-care today. This is a practical guide for truly sustainable self-care trans-lating to the care of others. Health systems would do well to implement such a program. We all stand to learn what is at the core of our doubts and discomfort. Digesting and internalizing this book, especially in the company of others, is truly the beginning of mastering joy in our work."
– **Lisa Prusak**, MD

"This book provides a life-changing roadmap for living your best life while caring for others, with the power to change the health care landscape." – **Laurel Ash, DNP, CNP, RN, College of St. Scholastica School of Nursing**

"This book is a tremendous resource, providing relevant, real-world exam-ples and advice for sustaining caring roles for both individuals and teams. The strategies outlined in each chapter are easy to follow. It is a guide to promote personal growth for creating the balance that we all so desperately crave and deserve." – **Shannon Kennelly**, DVM, Owner of Lakeville Family Pet Clinic, a small animal veterinary practice

"The unattended emotional toll of caregivers too often results in a stress-filled workplace, career-ending psychological trauma, or even suicide. This book will help you recognize, understand, and support a healthy, sustainable alternative." – **Mark Lavalier**, Firefighter

"*The world needs caregivers, and caregivers need this book, as did I. Using her own years of experience and research, Rev. Dr. Schuder has written an indispensable book with practical strategies, resources, and inspiration for achieving resilience and sustainability in personal and professional helping roles. Infused with hope and compassion, this book served as a supportive guide for me while caring for others.*" – **Diane Torvick**, Family Caregiver

"*This book is a powerful tool. If you read it and put it into practice, you will surely live with a better quality of life as an individual, as part of a family and a community. Karen provides a wisdom that helps people live more vibrantly.*" – **Miriam Sierra**, World Vision Honduras

"*Karen's insights and experience make this book a valuable guide for anyone in the helping professions. In the crisis-driven world of helping professions, this book will make the task more doable for any who take on the role of helper.*" – **David Spencer**, BA, MS, Retired Counselor in international and local schools and family and individual therapy

"*Dr. Schuder's work helped me shift my focus from making decisions based on approval to a purpose-driven outlook. This freed me to make a major career and life change that dramatically improved my resilience and ability to serve others while caring for my needs. Karen made me feel supported and valued at a time when I was experiencing burnout and exhaustion. She helped me see the value I bring to others because of the person I am, not just because of my role.*" – **Julie Knuths**, DNP, RN, PHN, Associate Professor and Chair, Department of Undergraduate Nursing, College of St. Scholastica

"*This deeply reflective book has the potential to benefit so many. What comes to mind, based on my experience in Africa and the Americas, are the frontline workers responding to humanitarian emergencies in their home countries: heroes who often need to process their own loss and grief and help their families through disaster while selflessly providing life-saving assistance to others."* – **Judith Anne Thimke**, Former UN World Food Programme Manager and Country Director

"If you hope to maintain a life or career of caregiving, understand the hazards along the way and embrace the personal survival skills this book will gift you." – **Charles Gallet**, Paramedic and CISD Leader

"During my many years of caregiving for multiple family members, I yearned for support and strategies to help me through the many challenges this presented. This book is exactly what I was looking for and needed. I'm grateful Karen saw the need for a book to help people navigate through this challenging journey that many of us face in our lives." – **Jan Arezzo**, Family Caregiver and Retired Educator

"I wish I had this workbook when I was a newly ordained woman in ministry. I wanted to do an excellent job helping people and the church. I worked too hard and eventually experienced burnout. If I had studied Resilient and Sustainable Caring, *I could have done a much better job managing the stress related to my position and caring for others. I wholeheartedly recommend this workbook to all caregivers!"* – **Rev. Sharon Johnson**, Retired Minister, Former Executive Presbyter

"This book guides you how to establish limits in caring for other people. This will allow you not only to prevent burnout, but live better professionally and personally, helping you remain resilient at your work in the long run. The concepts and skills have helped me deal with emotional people and find guidance based on my purpose." – **Merlyn Enrique Lara**, Medical Student

"Karen's comprehensive guide is based on research and lived experience. It is a welcome gift for helpers at any stage in their career, from starry-eyed beginners to exhausted senior staffers." – **Louise M. Beyea**, DVM, On-Call Private Practice Veterinarian for over thirty years

"This book is a thoughtful, concise resource for those in the helping professions to help themselves handle the stress of caring. It is especially helpful for those beginning or mid-career and provides practical tools that should be included in health professions' curricula. Don't wait until you're burned out to read this!" – **Kris Wegerson**, MD

"This book is a wonderful read! It provides insightful and encouraging advice on how to balance our various needs. I have benefited greatly from Karen's advice and thoughtful sharing of her experience. As an immigrant, full-time employee, daughter, wife, and mom of two young kids, I always strive to balance my work and my family and different cultures, as well as the needs of others and myself. Reading this book helps me find a better way to strike the balance in seeking true meaning in my life." – **Lin Xiu**, PhD, Associate Professor, Faculty of Human Resource Management, University of Minnesota Duluth

"Dr. Schuder provides welcoming space for personal reflection that thoughtfully influences sustainable practice for any caregiver." – **Lindsey Knox**, DVM, University of Minnesota College of Veterinary Medicine

"This book provides insight into a sensitive topic for caregivers as well as those who support them. Most people care deeply and want to help others, yet many times they question their own adequacy to assist others when confronted by what seems like an overwhelming situation. This book serves as a guide to validating those feelings as well as offering guidance and advice to build emotional-support capacities." – **Allen Lewis**, Fire Chief

RESILIENT AND SUSTAINABLE CARING

Your Guide To Thrive
While Helping Others

KAREN SCHUDER, EdD, MDiv, MAM

Whole Person Associates, Inc.
Duluth, MN

Published by Whole Person Associates, Inc.
101 West 2nd Street, Suite 203
Duluth, MN 55802-5004
USA

800-247-6789 Books@WholePerson.com WholePerson.com

RESILIENT AND SUSTAINABLE CARING:
YOUR GUIDE TO THRIVE WHILE HELPING OTHERS

Publishing and editorial team:
Author Bridge Media
Editorial Director: Helen Chang
Publishing Manager: Laurie Aranda

Whole Person Associates
Publisher: Jack Kosmach

Library of Congress Control Number: 2022943400

ISBN: 978-1-57025-372-0 -- paperback
978-1-57025-373-7 -- ebook

Ordering Information:
Quantity sales and special discounts are available on purchases by corporations,
associations, and others. For details, contact the publisher
at the address above.

DEDICATION

I dedicate this book to all the wonderful caregivers committed to making the world a healthier place.

I also dedicate this work to my wonderful husband, Steve, and children, Joshua, Caleb, and Sophia. You are truly the wind beneath my wings. All you do to make the world a better place lifts my heart and encourages me forward in the wonderful journey of helping others.

CONTENTS

Acknowledgments xiii

Introduction 1

1. **Start the Resilient and Sustainable Caring Journey** 9

   Thrive with a plan to: 1) strengthen your best, balanced self,
   2) decrease anxiety and increase emotional regulation, and
   3) expand support.

2. **Bring Out Your Strength with Core Values and Purpose** 25

   Increase resilience by identifying what's important and
   developing purpose that includes self-care.

3. **Promote Your Best, Balanced Self with Healthy Boundaries** 45

   Radiate goodness and help others do so while applying what's
   important to daily life.

4. **Foster Self-Compassion** 67

   Create emotional space by noticing personal suffering and
   responding with kindness.

5. **Decrease Anxiety** 91

   Nurture inner peace and reduce group anxiety by defusing
   emotional triggers and changing perspective.

6. **Deal with Conflict**...113

   Expand a capacity to create new possibilities while promoting helpful conflict habits.

7. **Recover from Loss** 135

   Find hope beyond loss to help others without taking on their grief.

8. **Lighten the Load with Resources** 155

   Empower healthy caring by redefining success to include use of resources and wise role changes.

9. **Grow Supportive Community**...177

   Expand community while nurturing connections and collective efforts encouraging balance.

10. **Thrive with Growing Strength and Resilience** 195

   Promote a joyful journey with strategies that positively change the world within and around you.

Appendix A: Suggested Reading List..203

Endnotes 209

About the Author 239

ACKNOWLEDGMENTS

As with so many of life's large endeavors, this book was made possible with the help of many wonderful people. I am so thankful for everyone who has provided support and wisdom over the years. Even if your name isn't on this page, know that I appreciate all of the people who touch my life journey. I would especially like to acknowledge and thank the following individuals:

The more than fifty people in personal and professional helping roles who took the time to share wisdom and stories with me. Whether in health care, nonprofit organizations, education, or family care—you are changing the world. You are an inspiration for me and many others. Keep on caring!

My husband, Steve, who has been my biggest support. You are my hero with your terrific legacy of caring for people and animals. My dear children, Sophia, Caleb, and Joshua. Your constant love and support have provided the courage to take this leap of faith. To my parents, Sandy and Dick, thanks for your love over the years. Laura, Beth, and Zack, I am thankful for your continued encouragement. This book is my gift to all of you with the hopes of returning some of the love and care you give so generously to me.

Family and friends who have taken the time to read early drafts and encourage me along the way. You are such a wonderful presence in my life. I especially want to acknowledge Sharon Johnson, MDiv;

Kris Wegerson, MD; Diane Torvick; Bonnie Keeling, MSW; Faris Keeling, MD; and Lin Xiu, PhD. Your insight and encouragement during the tough times have helped me more than you know.

Sociedad Amigos de los Ninos leadership and staff in Honduras, especially dear friends Sonia Erazo and Carolina Aguero. I am so thankful all of you are carrying Sor Maria Rosa's legacy of hope into the future.

Many Honduran friends, including Merlyn Enrique Lara and Javier Lara Cartagena, for helping me learn more about the beautiful people of Honduras.

Duluth Family Medicine Residency Program faculty and residents, especially Lisa Prusak, MD, for giving me insight into the challenges and delights of becoming a physician. I was touched by the kindness many of you so easily demonstrate.

College of St. Scholastica School of Nursing faculty, staff, and students, especially Laurel Ash, DNP; Julie Honey, DNP; and Julie Knuths, DNP, for inspiring me with your commitment to develop resilient, caring professionalism in a field that is vital for a healthy world and filled with incredible caring.

Helen Chang and Author Bridge Media. Your coaching and support have helped me to make a dream come true. Together we will promote resilient and sustainable caring in a world that so desperately needs people who can thrive while helping others.

INTRODUCTION

We Can Admit It—Helping Others Is Hard

The journey of helping others is adorned with beauty and littered with brokenness. Helping roles are filled with a grand mixture of hope, joy, sorrow, and frustration. Let's be honest—helping others can be exhausting. As caregivers, we take care of people and animals facing illness, trauma, and end of life. Sometimes we fall in bed with our clothes still on. We stop by fast-food restaurants to grab a bite while driving to the next appointment. We become so wrapped up in efforts to make the world a better place, we forget to take care of ourselves.

The sneaky message "self-care is selfish" slips into our busyness and becomes loud enough to make it even harder to take time for ourselves. We may feel guilty going on a walk when someone else needs help facing the end of life. Laughing with friends or playing with our dog seems out of place when we just left a family dealing with tragedy. We can have a hard time letting go of anger after someone said no to a great care plan. The world's suffering and brokenness bear witness to a desperate need for care and reveal why helping others is hard.

The organizations and societies we work for are supposed to promote helping efforts, but they actually create more challenges. Many organizations claim they value employees' well-being, but fail to back up their words with resources and policies. They validate skepticism about self-care with extensive demands and unrealistic expectations. As we give up more of ourselves, burnout, compassion fatigue, moral distress, and other challenges become part of the landscape.

Consider the backdrop of your helping roles. As you work to assist others, do you ever:

- Find it hard to take time to make a healthy meal or go on a walk?

- Feel like you are going to collapse each night?

- Experience relentless anxiety as you rush from patient to patient, face an unhappy family member, or deal with management?

- Want to be able to go home, read a book, talk with friends, and enjoy life, but can't stop thinking about a rude remark, an unsuccessful treatment, or tomorrow's busy schedule?

- Struggle to find delight in life's simple joys, like a child's silly joke or a dog's funny antics?

- Get overwhelmed with sadness after dealing with a terminal diagnosis or traumatic event?

- Think there are too many demands, but little help from management, colleagues, or family?

If you answered "YES!" to any of these statements, you are not alone.

We tend to think the challenges are unique to our profession or role, but there are many similarities across the spectrum of helpers. The caregiving landscape comprises some common elements: diminished time for self-care, increased pressures, lack of support, and continually growing needs. The emotional toll of suffering adds another layer to helping work. Grief and conflict also appear on caregiver journeys. You, along with many others, work hard, sincerely care, and struggle to find balance for personal wellness.

Check Out the Resilient and Sustainable Caring Journey

We can thrive and find great meaning as we help others, despite the challenges. Resilient, sustainable caring doesn't mean we won't face challenges, but it affirms the ability to help others while experiencing personal wellness and the strength to recover from difficulties. We not only bounce back from challenges, but become stronger and have the confidence to handle difficult situations.

Thoughts about the day's tasks energize us like a fresh-brewed cup of coffee, rather than leave us feeling empty. We can make tough decisions and hold people's hands during traumatic times, and then let go of the strain and embrace the goodness of life. We respond to loss and trauma with self-compassion and rely on a strong support system. We can laugh with our children and play with the dog even after a tough day. A resilient and sustainable journey is one we can thrive on and enjoy over time.

Resilient, sustainable caring doesn't just happen, but requires intentionality. This book provides guidance and practical strategies to thrive while helping others. Grounded in values and purpose, we promote our best, balanced self. We also decrease anxiety and increase supportive community. All of this means we journey longer and feel happier in our personal and professional helping roles. As we make the path of helping others wide enough to include self-care, we see more beauty along the way and recover more quickly from challenges.

Caregiver resilience and sustainability is not a solo adventure. We influence and are influenced by the people whose journeys intersect with our own. Helping work often involves families and teams, so we will consider ways to increase group resilience and sustainability. *Resilient and Sustainable Caring* is grounded in research, social theories, and decades of experience to provide sound, practical guidance.

I want to help you thrive on the goodness of what you are doing. We can experience the joys of life even in the midst of emotional extremes—navigate the turns, bumps, and detours of caregiving with practical concepts and tools. Whether you are in a professional or personal role, this book will help you:

- Find healthy balance between personal care, relationships, and caregiving.

- Discover and benefit from an abundance of resources.

- Expand support within and outside of helping environments.

- Know when and how to make role changes to revitalize motivation.

- Learn from challenges and mistakes for wiser, more self-compassionate caregiving.

- Deal with conflict and loss in ways that promote growth, rather than burnout.

- Decrease anxiety's toll and see more of the positives in helping others.

- Offer yourself the kindness you so willingly give to others.

- Increase purpose and peace that endures beyond suffering.

- Experience more joy and goodness even after exposure to trauma.

- Promote authenticity and courage so you can care for others with heart rather than fear.

- Delight in who you are while embracing vulnerabilities and strengths.

Even when challenged, you can find nourishment and increase resilience for the path ahead. Thank you for taking the journey to help others in our beautiful, mixed-up world. You give and receive a wonderful gift while shaping life with the simple yet profound concept of care. Together, we can make sure the path we travel leads to a healthier world for all.

Know Where Resilient and Sustainable Caring Comes From

I have walked, stumbled, and danced along a caregiver path for decades. I learned the principles and strategies in *Resilient and Sustainable Caring* while helping people in times of trauma and supporting other caregivers in healthcare, advocacy groups, and family roles. My quest for resilience and sustainability began while working with severely, multiply handicapped preschool children and their families. I loved being with the children, yet my heart broke often from the suffering and loss involved. Rewarding—yes; sustainable—no.

The need for resilience and sustainability became even more pronounced in my later helping work. As pastor and community advocate, I helped people enduring deep mental illness, escaping from abuse, recovering from deep loss, and facing end of life. I also have led a wellness program for family-physician residents, engaged in ongoing work in Honduras, and provided support for staff at our family-owned veterinary clinic. Helping others has given and demanded much.

My journey helping people with such a wide variety of needs included deep questions, such as: How can I enjoy the blessings of my life after exposure to so much suffering? Given my desire to make the world a healthier place, how can I find energy when the needs and lack of progress seem overwhelming? How can I justify self-care when I'm addressing needs that seem so dire? I have sought out theories, research, and wisdom to answer such questions, to promote resilience and sustainability.

I am excited to share a multitude of helpful discoveries. My doctoral research on ethics and professional development neatly aligns with literature on countering burnout and compassion fatigue. My work and training in countering compassion fatigue, conflict mediation, grief, leadership development, organizational culture, and cultural differences provides a solid foundation for my program. *Resilient and Sustainable Caring* represents more than thirty years of learning and experience on how to navigate the demanding journey of helping others.

The wisdom I share comes from a wide range of sources, including a wonderful variety of caregivers. I have interviewed more than fifty individuals with experience in North and Central America, Africa, Europe, Asia, and Australia. They represent family caregivers, healthcare providers (human and veterinary), first responders, educators, clergy, and nonprofit advocates. You can read pieces of their experience and wisdom in the quotes labeled *Voices from the Field* found in this book.

Helpers in different roles have responded with excitement to my resilience and sustainability program. Medical residents openly talked about vulnerabilities and promoted self-care. Family caregivers gratefully looked at common challenges. Nurses energetically responded when discovering ways to navigate difficult scenarios. Honduran professionals eagerly discussed concepts promoting sustainability. Veterinary staff excitedly learned about fostering self-compassion. Enthusiasm from many committed helpers fuels the work behind this book.

My work is successful because I provide fresh ways for us to understand ourselves, along with practical tools promoting immediate sustainability. I use proven theories and ancient wisdom to build resilience and counter challenges such as compassion fatigue and burnout. Family Systems Theory is especially helpful as it provides important perspective on individuality and relationships. Concepts offer strategies to maintain a sense of self and decrease anxiety while being connected with others. You will experience "Yes! It's not just me" and "aha!" moments as you read this book and apply ideas, stories, and strategies specific to helping roles.

Let's Thrive While Helping Others

The resilient, sustainable journey begins with bringing out the strength we have within. Clarification of purpose and small changes in how we understand ourselves will transform life experiences and help us respond with fortitude. Thoughtful activities will help us discover a wonderful depth of hope, courage, wisdom, and self-compassion. We function from the best part of who we are when grounded in important principles and purpose.

With greater self-awareness, we are more able to promote peace—both internal and external. Choosing from a supply of skills, we will build resilience, decrease anxiety, and face difficult life situations with grace. We will loosen the grip of anxiety, conflict, and loss while connecting deeply with others. We can be at our best, especially when there are challenges.

Take this journey to promote your best, balanced self and help others do so too. Go through the book with colleagues or friends using the discussion questions at the end of each chapter. Honest conversations about challenges and strategies are a great way to develop a supportive community with other helpers.

We do make a difference as we help. We can find immense joy and meaning while navigating the difficult. Resilience helps us bounce back and thrive, not just stumble along. We can promote vibrant caring with ideas, skills, and strategies from *Resilient and Sustainable Caring*.

The time you take to help yourself is a gift for you and each person whose life you touch. Are you ready to increase balance and joy while helping others? If so, let's begin the wonderful journey to greater resilience and sustainability.

Chapter 1

START THE RESILIENT AND SUSTAINABLE CARING JOURNEY

*You can promote resilience and sustainability to thrive amid
the challenges of helping others. You are worth the effort
it takes to do this.*

Know You Aren't Alone

We cannot escape the realities of our helping work. We show kindness only to have it sometimes rewarded with rudeness. We fall in bed exhausted each day, and someone says, "You need to work harder." We beautifully explain a need for change only to have others say no. Helping others can be like a wild roller-coaster ride, moving between the emotions of delights and challenges.

We caregivers hang on during the challenges, holding people in the midst of trauma, and then struggle to let go of their suffering after we leave work. We go beyond expectations to heal, only to be left with feelings of helplessness when outcomes don't change. This is true whether we are nurses, physicians, family caregivers, veterinarians, first responders, clergy, counselors, advocates, educators, or any other helping role.

If you struggle to find balance, you are among the many caregivers who put energy, heart, and soul into helping others while longing for personal wellness and resilience. As people who care, we are exposed to a wide range of demands. Even with the most virtuous of intentions, our efforts bump up against the world's brokenness. We are exposed to some of the harshest realities and can feel powerless. Whatever helping role you are in, you journey with people all over the world who can relate to the challenges you face.

One message I hope to impart is that everyone struggles at times. When you struggle, this does not mean you are deficient, but that you are human. I also want to communicate clearly that you are not alone. People in helping roles around the world understand how hard caring can be. You can find support from an array of caregivers with similar stories.

We tend to think challenges we face are unique to our profession or role. However, many challenges cross the spectrum of people helping others. For example, a Centers for Disease Control and Prevention (CDC) study showed increased psychological distress and suicidal ideation among veterinarians.[1] Researchers attributed this to compassion fatigue resulting from increased pressures, suffering, and loss.

I focused on helping people understand and counter compassion fatigue in response to this study. After hearing about my work, first responders, dentists, physicians, nurses, and family caregivers energetically responded, saying, "We also need that!" Caregivers in personal and professional roles face common challenges and share a need to improve role sustainability.

Research confirms our intuition that more is needed to promote sustainability among helping roles. An American Medical Association

(AMA) survey of physicians showed a 42 percent burnout rate.[2] Other studies revealed that more than half of US physicians and nurses surveyed experience burnout.[3] Burnout occurs across helping roles, and it's not the only challenge facing helpers.

The American Psychological Association (APA) acknowledged the prevalence of compassion fatigue among mental health-care providers.[4] Researchers in India concluded dentists are prone to burnout, depression, and anxiety.[5] A survey of first responders revealed higher rates of suicidal thoughts.[6] You can easily find articles about burnout and other challenges among helpers like educators and family caregivers.

Demands are taking a toll on helpers globally. I have listened to wonderful caregivers from five continents share the difficulties they have encountered. Many can echo what Jose, a Honduran physician, said, "I love my work, but it is so exhausting. There are so many of us who don't know what to do to make it better. Rates of burnout and suicide are high." To work in the midst of suffering is to experience the best and worst the world has to offer. Helping others is among the most rewarding and most demanding of journeys.

We have to make it more sustainable, because caregivers embody one of the most honorable, and necessary, activities. Virginia Held wrote, "Care is probably the most deeply fundamental value . . . There can be no justice without care, however, for without care no child would survive and there would be no persons to respect."[7]

The importance and challenges of helping others inspired me to develop a sustainable way to care. Our work can be hard, but it is vital to the world's well-being. Despite the difficulties, we can thrive while bringing care into the world.

SEE COMMON CHALLENGES: FROM BURNOUT AND COMPASSION FATIGUE TO IMPOSTER SYNDROME, YOU ARE NOT ALONE

The following descriptions provide basic explanations to promote awareness and identification with others who face similar challenges. It is important to note the descriptions do not give enough information to make diagnoses. That is something only qualified professionals should do. I wholeheartedly encourage you to use resources such as a therapist or counselor to help prevent or recover from challenges.

Burnout: Burnout is a state of exhaustion caused by involvement with emotionally demanding situations over a long-term period.[8] It is the chronic condition of perceived demands being greater than available resources.[9]

Primary and Secondary Trauma: Trauma is an extreme form of stress after a distressing event. The reaction is so strong that typical recovery responses don't reestablish life as it was before.[10]

- Primary trauma occurs when we personally experience or witness an event that evokes fear and helplessness.[11]

- Secondary trauma refers to accumulated stress resulting from exposure to other people's traumas.[12] This vicarious trauma shifts our worldview after we're exposed through images or stories.[13]

Compassion Fatigue: A synergistic interaction between primary trauma, secondary trauma, and burnout over time may lead to compassion fatigue.[14] Repeated exposure to other people's traumas, combined with a perceived lack of resources and primary trauma built up over time, can take a toll on personal well-being and motivation.

Moral Distress: Moral distress occurs when individuals are called to act in ways that oppose their personal values and morals.[15] This can be due to policies or organizational expectations that oppose what we believe is right. We pay a price when encountering situations that violate our fundamental beliefs of what is right and wrong.

Imposter Syndrome: This is the feeling that you do not have what is needed for your role, accompanied by the fear of being unmasked as a fraud.[16] Imposter feelings are common among high achievers during times of professional transitions.[17] Perfectionism, along with thinking one needs to succeed without help, contributes to the sense of not fitting a role.

Keep in mind that burnout, trauma, compassion fatigue, moral distress, and imposter syndrome have names because many people have experienced them. These challenges can have physical, emotional, social, behavioral, and work-related implications. Loss of ideals, decreased sense of accomplishment, and feelings of isolation are among the most dangerous. Struggles we experience point to a reality we cannot escape: helping people amid difficult circumstances takes a toll. If you are having a hard time, remember you are not alone.

If at any point you feel you are in danger of harming yourself or being harmed by someone else, please be wise and seek immediate assistance. There is always hope. Sometimes we need others to help us see that. We all are human and need help at times. A point of utmost importance: You are worth caring about.

Look Beyond Burnout . . . My Story

My conviction that we can thrive while helping others has developed over a long, difficult journey. I entered a helping career believing that love can conquer all, but discovered a lot of brokenness may be involved. Little did I know when I accepted the pastor position at two small, rural churches that my life and profession were on a collision course that would leave me on the floor weeping.

Lake Church and First Church congregations had a long history of conflict. Lake Church resembled a Northwoods cabin, with pine walls and stained-glass-window images of birch trees. Most of the church members had retired and moved to their cabins, where they could fish and escape busy city traffic. Lake Church was only a twenty-minute drive from First Church, but a world away.

First Church's white building sat in the middle of a small town with three other buildings. Most members grew up in the area and tried to make a living on small dairy farms. Two tables filled the social hall, one for the men and the other for the women. The first time I approached the men's table, there was a collective breath as I sat down to hear some of their stories. I worked hard to let the people of First Church and Lake Church know I cared about them.

I visited with people in their homes to learn about their families and said prayers with them after surgeries. I listened to stories about loved ones who had died and celebrated births of their grandchildren. About a year after starting as pastor, I became pregnant, and we welcomed our daughter Sophia into the world. Steve and I navigated the challenges of a young family and demanding jobs. I returned to work tired, but ready.

First Church's women held a baby shower to welcome Sophie with pastel blankets, knitted sweaters, and a handmade cradle. I was completely unaware of issues until someone said, "Lake Church is caus-ing problems again." I assured them I would talk with church leaders and work on any issues. Leaders from Lake Church said nothing was wrong, but each Sunday I saw a growing number of hate-filled faces.

I eventually learned a member of Lake Church had talked with members of both congregations, explaining that I should not be their pastor. Gossip spread like wildfire. Statements included: "She just had a baby and shouldn't be working," "We can't rely on her," and "Her husband has a good job, we shouldn't have to pay her so much." I was paid less than minimum wage and had not missed a day before maternity leave.

During Christmas celebrations, I was trying to understand and dismantle the conflict. I put on a good face, but my stomach was knotted and I wanted to cry. I had to convince myself to get up on Sunday mornings and drive to Lake Church, where I knew I would face hateful stares again.

Shortly after Christmas, we learned that my mother-in-law, Ruth, was critically ill with an aggressive form of strep. Over the next few weeks, my husband and I divided our time between home and the hospital. We slept on chairs in the hospital waiting room and took turns to be with Ruth, who was on life support. I felt overwhelmed by responsibilities and powerlessness.

On the weekends, I led worship services, meetings, and pastoral visits. Eventually, discontent at Lake Church erupted at a contract meeting. Some members yelled accusations such as, "She's trying to take advantage of us!" Individuals I thought would support me were silent. One person said, "What we are doing to her is wrong." I drove home stunned, shaking, and racing through the darkness to get to my safe place and safe people.

Our house was empty, and I didn't know where Steve and the kids were. My professional hopes were dashed. I felt like a failure, unworthy of being supported. Idealism was cast into the wind, and it seemed as though all the good things I had done were worthless. I fell on our living room floor and wept. My bones ached and my stomach hurt. I have never felt so betrayed or lonely as I did that day. I was utterly exhausted, but couldn't find rest.

I was tormented by whether to continue as the congregations' pastor. Thoughts of being at Lake Church made my heart race and palms sweat. I cried and prayed a lot. Ruth miraculously recovered, and this provided a renewed sense of hope. One day, the emotional fog lifted, and I knew it was okay to leave. I can see now that was the moment healing began, although all I could feel was pain.

This painful experience inspired me to get serious about finding more sustainable ways to care. The long, slow climb to wellness included time hugging my children and Steve, and meeting with a spiritual director. Friends and mentors also provided valuable perspective. A spark to promote self-care while helping others was kindled. I worked hard to heal and be my best, balanced self for the sake of my family.

I thought I would never be able to work as a pastor again, but never say never. With much support, I did say yes and was pastor to a wonderful congregation for twelve years. Over the years, I continually sought ways to care and lead while promoting personal wellness. Self-awareness became integral to building resilience and sustainability.

I worked hard to remain grounded in what was important. Healthy boundaries and self-compassion became part of my journey. I pursued learning opportunities to expand my abilities for dealing with difficult situations, such as loss and conflict. My role often involved participation in various colleague and community groups that provided support.

My journey continues to include challenges and suffering, but the beauty and joy of care shines brighter than anything else. I can see the hard parts of helping people and organizations, but awareness of meaningful experiences and relationships shines brighter. Our caring roles are filled with the mix of life and can be sustainable. We can bounce back from challenges to face the journey of helping others with greater strength and wisdom.

Create a Resilience and Sustainability Plan

No matter where you are in your journey, you can see and do things to experience the joy, fulfillment, and camaraderie of caregiving. I know how tiring and overwhelming being a helper can feel. I also know the benefits can outweigh challenges and bumps in the road. We all are touched by suffering, but we can influence how it shapes our lives. We can do more than overcome the brokenness behind suffering. I am excited to share what I have learned through experience, research, and theory. We can thrive while promoting balance and resilience.

You will increase resilience and balance so you can thrive while moving through *Resilient and Sustainable Caring*. Three components are woven throughout: (1) strengthen your best, balanced self, (2) decrease anxiety and increase emotional regulation, and 3) expand support. All three overlap and work to increase resilience and sustainability. Explanations, stories, and tools can help you apply concepts right now. Approaches for fostering resilience in others also are provided. My hope is to help you help yourself while you help others. That's a lot of help!

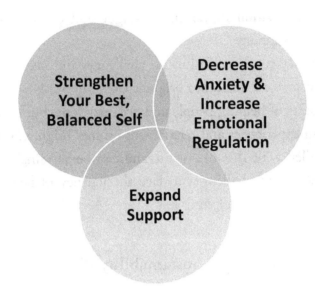

Part 1: Strengthen Your Best, Balanced Self

Chapters:

- Bring Out Your Strength with Core Values and Purpose.
- Promote Your Best, Balanced Self with Healthy Boundaries.
- Foster Self-Compassion.

We start with strengthening the best part of who we are, the core values and purpose behind wanting to help others. When we guide our path purposefully with what we consider important, we can be at our best, balanced self even in the midst of storms. Knowing what is important, and responding in ways that reflect basic values and purpose, are central to resilience and sustainability. As Nietzsche wrote, "(One) who has a why to live for can bear almost any how."[18]

When we live in ways aligned with core values and beliefs, we are not tossed around as much. Knowing our purpose shifts focus from unhelpful anxieties, fears, and pressures to what really matters. Your best, balanced self is not the perfect you in a perfect world, but the *vibrant you* successfully managing all your roles. Being our best, balanced self involves living in healthy ways that reflect important values and purpose. As we identify what this means, we create a valuable map for the journey.

Once we understand how to live as our best, balanced self, we can promote healthy boundaries that keep us on a sustainable path. Limits designating what we are and aren't responsible for help us create harmony between care of self and others. Emotional boundaries are among the most difficult to understand, but are vital to sustainability. Once we identify our emotional responsibilities, we can discover ways to be in the midst of suffering without getting caught up in other people's emotional storms. We are affected by suffering, but can influence how it marks our journey.

When we feel suffering's impact, we can respond with self-compassion to promote wellness. We are encouraged to be compassionate toward others, but seldom emboldened to offer it to ourselves. Self-compassion honors our common humanity with kindness and provides a hopeful "you can handle this." It counters perfectionism and unrealistic demands. Forgiveness, a piece of compassion, enables us to keep moving on our journey after falling short of expectations. Self-compassion provides a life jacket when it feels like the waters are too stormy.

As we strengthen our best, balanced self with important values and purpose, healthy boundaries, and self-compassion, we step closer to a balanced journey. The next step is increasing our ability to regulate anxiety and emotions. Inner calm gives us the ability to stay on course and enjoy the journey, even when storms erupt.

Part 2: Decrease Anxiety and Increase Emotional Regulation

Chapters:

- Decrease Anxiety.

- Deal with Conflict.

- Recover from Loss.

Anxiety at healthy levels pushes us to be more productive and proactive. Unfortunately, it is too easy to get caught up in unsustainable levels of chronic anxiety. Bonnie, a social worker, discovered this after having a heart attack. When her cardiologist asked, "Do you have any stress in your life?" she immediately responded, "No!" After thinking about it, Bonnie realized she answered too quickly. She explained, "When I looked at the clipboard with a list of everything I was doing, I felt dizzy. It felt like the world was spinning out of control."

No matter how smart or skilled we are, the world's endless demands and busyness takes a toll. The good news is we can change how much anxiety we experience. Differentiating our emotions from those of others lies at the heart of this work. Greater self-knowledge helps us identify and change emotional triggers to decrease reactivity. Small changes in how we perceive ourselves alter how we experience pressures. For example, as we turn our focus to being purpose driven rather than praise motivated, we are influenced less by other people's anxiety.

We can promote inner peace through mindful activities, calming exercises, and spiritual nourishment. Being calm within loosens anxiety's grip on our lives. Internal peace can help us face life challenges with greater integrity and wisdom.

Conflict and loss are among the most difficult life challenges, but they don't need to bring our journey to a stop. Proactive work and skills help us influence their impact on our own lives and those we interact with. We may not be able to remove conflict or loss from life, but we can respond in ways that reduce anxiety and promote sustainability.

We also have the choice to increase or decrease the anxiety spreading through families, teams, and organizations. As tricky as relationships can be, they are an incredible source of resilience and sustainability. The more we intentionally develop resources and foster nourishing relationships, the better we can deal with difficult interactions on our journey and help others do so on their journeys. Let's harness the energy so it helps us move forward rather than knocks us over.

Part 3: Expand Support

Chapters:
- Lighten the Load with Resources.
- Grow Supportive Community.

We often have more resources than we are aware of. An array of strategies, relationships, opportunities, and activities can help us find energy and support for our journey of care. Once we know available resources, we have to take the next step of allowing ourselves to use them. Often, this involves seeing success differently and dealing with silencers so we can talk about challenges. We may find and provide safe support with intentional efforts to develop deeper connections.

Meaningful connections affirm and validate who we are. Family, friends, colleagues, and others who provide support help us keep the bounce in our step. Professional providers can equip us with important objectivity and tools no matter where we are on the journey of helping others. Healthy relationships add much needed perspective and care, but also require intentional efforts to develop.

We can discover myriad ways to nurture meaningful relationships and opportunities to share. After intentionally being grounded in what is important and decreasing anxiety, we find more energy to invest in deeper connections. We also are more likely to use the available resources that provide nourishment and guidance. We will consider ways to develop a vast resource network and overcome the silencers that make it hard to share authentically. Groups nurturing authenticity and care are truly a gift.

Community can be bigger than we think it is, so we may benefit from looking at ways to expand connections. A variety of creative tasks provide ideas for how to grow our support field. Resilience and balance in teams is not a solo act. As we work to increase resilience and sustainability for ourselves, we positively influence others in our lives—family, teams, and organizations. We caregivers can provide valuable support to each other.

Always remember that you have support. Know also that your best, most important source of support is . . . you.

Be Your Best Advocate

As we learn how to be our own best resource, we can support others more effectively. If there is anything you take from this book, I hope it is this: you are worth caring about. You can find hope and people who care about you. This book is based on theory and research, but does not replace support from mental health-care providers. If at any time you find it hard to function, please talk to a professional counselor. On this journey of helping others, you are your most important advocate.

You will get the most out of this book by reading through from the beginning. Chapters 2 and 3 are especially foundational. They establish the groundwork for your guide to thrive with resilient, sustainable caring. Concepts progress with each chapter and include a variety of practical strategies. The book is formatted in short sections, so you can read in brief or extended sessions. Use the concepts and tasks to create a guide to thrive. Once read, you can return to *Resilient and Sustainable Caring* as a resource for ongoing guidance.

Study alone or with a group to promote meaningful discussions about the challenges and joys of helping others. For every challenge we face, many people are struggling with the same hurdles. We are never alone in facing the challenges of helping roles, and together we can promote authentic support and validate the blessings of self-care.

"Self-care is never a selfish act," wrote Parker Palmer. "It is simply good stewardship of the only gift I have, the gift I was put on earth to offer others. Anytime we can listen to true self and give the care it requires, we do it not only for ourselves, but for the many others whose lives we touch."[19]

How we treat ourselves affects our ability to care for others. We can promote wellness and model healthy caring to future generations. Just as important, we will positively influence the teams and systems we work with to promote resilient, sustainable caring.

You can turn the hills into bumps with self-care. You are worth the effort. Resilience and balance will help you enjoy life, especially as you take on the journey of helping others. Now that you have an idea of the map for resilient and sustainable caring, get ready to strengthen your best, balanced self. Embrace the best part of who you are. Promote personal wellness and thrive while changing the world with care. The next step awaits you!

Chapter 2

Bring Out Your Strength with Core Values and Purpose

We increase sustainability by being purpose driven rather than praise motivated.

Strengthen Yourself with Purpose

Purpose is powerful. We can find great strength and resilience through purpose, but only if we know what that purpose is. When we lack clarity, it's easy to be driven and drained by the pressures coming at us. I experienced this many times over the years, but especially after the 2001 terrorist attacks.

In some ways the world stopped on September 11, yet in other ways it seemed to spin out of control. I was solo pastor of a congregation at the time and had begun the morning by visiting Ken, a soft-spoken man struggling with the recent move to a care center. When I arrived, he quickly muted the morning news show and greeted me with a sad smile. After pleasantries, Ken informed me he had just been diagnosed with advanced stages of cancer.

As Ken shared this sad news, an image on the television caught my eye: a plane flying into a World Trade Center tower. I tried to focus on supporting him but found my gaze wandering back to the disturbing images. Just after leaving Ken, I learned about the terrorist attacks unfolding. Collective and individual grief was overwhelming.

I thrive on helping people during difficult times, but this occasion was touched with personal grief as well. The days, weeks, and months after were filled with people who needed support. Helping individuals with deep needs was added to ongoing organizational demands, care of our young family, and support of our business. As you most likely know, times of intense emotion and anxiety can leave us feeling rudderless in a stormy world.

Lack of clarity regarding values and purpose makes us more vulnerable to the volatile forces of our struggling world. I had a sense of what I believed, but during times of intense pressure this melted into the background. As much as I tried to leave work at work, the effects of a challenging job and world seeped into my personal life, increasing stress, guilt, and exhaustion. I knew this wasn't sustainable. I yearned to become more grounded in what I felt was important, not tossed around by growing anxieties.

"If one doesn't know to which port one is sailing, no wind is favorable," noted the ancient philosopher Seneca. Without a destination in mind, we can't tell a good wind from a bad wind and are moved by the whim of whatever winds are blowing. Important principles, including purpose, help us know the good winds. Clear understanding of important beliefs, values, and purpose provides a vision of our destination and helps us tap into forces that move us forward.

Your core beliefs and purpose can be the most powerful source of guidance and resilience, but only if you know what they are. Articulation of core beliefs creates a map for your journey that fosters confidence to navigate turns and hurdles with determination. The ideals drawing you to help other people provide the strength to thrive. I am thankful for the sense of purpose leading you to care for others. I want to help you increase sustainability by using your most valuable resource—you.

Let's venture into bringing out the best, strongest part of you: your core beliefs, values, virtues, and purpose. Part of this work includes balancing your purpose to promote personal well-being. Also, teams can increase resilience and sustainability through unified purpose. Core values and purpose provide guidance for the journey amid a variety of pressures. Or, to use Seneca's analogy, they define the port you are trying to get to and a rudder to steer you in the right direction, no matter what winds are blowing.

///

Resilience at Work: Imagine . . .

You face a variety of challenges that sometimes feel overwhelming. Expectations pull you in different directions, and on occasion you encounter suffering that hits harder than expected. At times you want to scream, run, or hide, but instead you remember what is really important. You take a deep breath to slow down and think about your purpose. Grounded in core beliefs, you face challenges with optimism, process how to best respond, and give yourself space to reenergize. You know the journey can be hard, but also filled with meaning and goodness.

///

Decrease Pressures with Authenticity

Ongoing pressures from a variety of directions can challenge your efforts to help others sustainably—in part because pressures can make it difficult to be authentic and provide self-care. As you work toward being who you feel called to be, do you ever feel stretched or sidelined by:

- A continued need to prove yourself?
- Efforts to keep everyone happy?
- Fears of making a mistake?
- Desires to fit in?
- Unrealistic expectations?
- An atmosphere of negativity and anxiety?
- An intolerance of diversity?
- Stereotypes?

Such pressures drain energy as they pull us away from living in ways aligned with important values. They can make us feel as though we are chasing an ideal that keeps slipping away, because anxiety gets in the way.

Our journey will always include forces tugging us in different directions. Many pressures come from our need for connection with others.[1] We all face a tug and pull between being distinct individuals while wanting to be accepted by others. We cannot escape both needs. However, we can decrease the pressures of belonging when we function more from well-thought-out values, beliefs, and purpose.[2]

As we define what is important, we move core beliefs to a central part of life. We function from the best, most mature part of ourselves.[3] This helps us differentiate from other people's feelings, perspectives, and anxieties. Self-differentiation, a Family Systems Theory concept, involves being able to define our own life goals and values separate from the pressures of others.[4] Increased self-differentiation reduces the anxiety caused by our need for acceptance, so we are more able to live authentically and allow others to do so as well.

Voices from the Field: Ground yourself in what's important.

"It's really important to know your values when leading teams. When we are grounded in what's important, we can stand up for what we believe. If you don't know who you are, how can you help your crew know who they are? If we are making life-and-death decisions for other people, we need to know where we are coming from and what those decisions are based on." Lisa, Firefighter, United States

---

Self-differentiation expands our capacity to be around other people's anxieties without absorbing them or changing for them.[5] As we function based on core principles, we increase the ability to think rationally, regulate emotions, problem solve creatively, and connect with others in healthy ways.[6] We can compassionately care while honoring the truth that we do not need to carry others' emotions. We embrace what is key to who we are and become more purpose driven.

A purpose-driven journey creates a more solid path than one determined by pressures, anxieties, and emotions in a constantly fluctuating world.[7] Purpose orientation promotes resilience and counters challenges such as moral distress, burnout, and compassion fatigue. Functioning in ways aligned with personal beliefs encourages well-being.[8] It is more energizing to face each day with known direction rather than reacting to the unknown. A clear sense of purpose helps us make decisions we feel good about and fosters positive perspectives.

> *Your purpose in life is to find your purpose and give your whole heart and soul to it.* —Buddha

Build Purpose-Driven Resilience

A purpose-driven mindset positively affects how we see our work. Italian psychologist Roberto Assagioli wrote a parable about the power of purpose that involved three men building a medieval cathedral.[9] All three men were stonecutters, but each saw his work very differently.

When asked, the first stonecutter responded bitterly and described the monotonous task of cutting blocks. With a sense of doom, he noted that he would be doing this the rest of his life. The second individual described the task and explained with warmth how he was providing for his family. The third stonecutter responded with joy, sharing how he was privileged to participate in building a great cathedral that would be a source of hope for thousands of years.

"Competence may bring us satisfaction," wrote physician Rachel Naomi Remen. "Finding meaning in a familiar task often allows us to go beyond this and find in the most routine of tasks a deep sense of joy and even gratitude."[10] How we see our role and context determines whether our work will deplete or nourish us.[11] As we live in ways that reflect core beliefs, we discover the power of being part of a larger purpose.[12]

Purpose increases inspiration, courage, and resilience.[13] In *Man's Search for Meaning*, Viktor Frankl recounted experiences as a prisoner in World War II concentration camps.[14] Prisoners who couldn't see a life purpose lost hope. They refused to get dressed in the morning or talk with others during social times, and instead silently laid on the threadbare mattresses. Their health quickly declined. Those who found purpose in helping others by sharing their last piece of bread or giving words of encouragement were more likely to survive.

Voices from the Field: Find deeper meaning.

"I found I need to understand my purpose as being much bigger than the work environment. Helping people is bigger than where you work. There is a deeper meaning to what we do than what our contract spells out, and some of the most important rewards are not financial." Jay, Physician, United States

---

We often think we know our purpose and what is important to us, but until we actually write it down it remains something lurking on the periphery. Without clarity, important beliefs at the core of who we are tug at our conscience rather than guide us on the best path. The core of who we are is based on fundamental beliefs, values, virtues, and purpose. Consider core concepts to clarify personal purpose. We all are influenced by other people's beliefs, and it is vital to tease through those influences to discern our own.

Acknowledge the influence of others, but clearly identify your own beliefs, values, virtues, and purpose. Understand what makes you unique and can drive your journey forward. This work of defining self can help you walk alongside others without getting stuck on someone else's journey. Defining what is important helps us know good winds from bad winds.

DEFINE AND ARTICULATE WHAT'S IMPORTANT

Beliefs: Describe the belief systems, events, and individuals that have shaped how you see the world. Examples include culture, faith background, life-changing experiences, and influential people. This work can help you think about the beliefs you have been exposed to and what to embrace, reshape, or let go of. Identify why you believe what you believe, and you will know better what to embrace as your own.

Values: Define the most important values you want to guide your decisions and actions. As you think about what is significant enough to shape how you use time, energy, and finances, determine the key value involved. Core values should be bigger than a profession or role and apply to every life context.

Important Virtues: Determine the virtues that stand out as especially important. Our values may include virtues, but there is a distinction between the two. Virtues are qualities leading to moral excellence and collective well-being.[15] Examples of virtues include compassion, courage, creativity, generosity, gratitude, honesty, hope, humility, joyfulness, kindness, love, loyalty, patience, peace, respect, and wisdom. We can attain happiness and positively impact the world when we practice virtues, but we need to be intentional about doing so.[16]

Integration of all virtues is encouraged, but our souls sing louder as we foster personally important virtues. Consider the behaviors you believe are important for healthy living and identify the virtues they represent. Another approach is to consider actions that bother you. Behaviors that push your buttons typically reveal a violation of an important virtue. Identifying important values and virtues provides guidance to living in vibrant ways.

Strengths: A strength is the skill, talent, and knowledge you use consistently with high levels of success.[17] In determining your strengths, don't get stuck on comparisons to other people, as this rarely brings out the best in us. Others may have similar talents, but this does not negate the contribution of your strengths. Be creative as you think about strengths and acknowledge those outside of role-specific skill sets.

Technical knowledge and skills are important but don't sum up what makes people proficient. Even individuals with the most advanced technical skills and knowledge need other strengths to succeed. Try to recognize the array of strengths you bring to helping others. You are the only person who needs to see this list, so don't be shy or stingy. When struggling, review the list to gain perspective and confidence. People who work from their strengths are more effective at tasks and roles and find greater satisfaction even amid challenges.[18]

Growth Areas: Honest self-awareness goes beyond strengths to include acknowledgment of weaknesses. While greater focus on strengths provides positives, we also need to understand how we can grow. Seeing our weaknesses honors our humanness and provides wisdom as to how we can best focus self-development efforts. Create a list that doesn't overwhelm you, but energizes you to change and expand. Just like the natural world around us, we are more fully alive when we are growing.

Motivation and Inspiration: What gets you excited about the work you do? What cause, activity, or concept makes your heart beat a little faster when you talk about it? Identify what fires you up, and use that to bring a healthy passion to life. Name the driving factors that led you to your helping roles. Whether you are new or experienced, the passion leading you is a vital part of resilience. Claim it and reclaim it for years to come. Remind yourself daily why you do what you do, and dedicate time to nourish this motivation.

Nourish your body, mind, and soul to build resilience, enjoy life, and pursue purpose. After you consider core concepts, you will possess a clearer understanding of self and increase your ability to make decisions based on what is important rather than external pressures. From this self-awareness, you can more readily discern your life direction and develop a purpose statement. Your purpose statement will remind you what is important and help you navigate the intersections, hurdles, and turns in your journey.

Voices from the Field: Know where you stand.

"We need to have awareness of our own values and beliefs. They are going to be different from others', and that's okay. You need to know where to draw the line in the sand when confronted with difficult situations. Values and beliefs may change when you want, but they should never change because you feel forced to." Raye, Veterinarian, United States

---

Clarify Purpose

We are less likely to get derailed by other people's purpose when we know our own. I saw this on a microfinance trip in Honduras. We gathered around a brick oven fueled by sticks as the scent of baking cookies filled the air. Four women with flour scattered on their clothing proudly showed us how they were changing the rural Honduran community with their blossoming bakery. A few men observed from the sidelines as our group from the United States asked questions.

Most of the trip participants brought a corporate mindset and operated with a perspective focused on money. So, when one community member explained she sold milk to a neighbor for less money to help the individual, a microfinance team member had difficulty grasping the social implications. He responded, "But if you can sell it for more, why don't you?" He missed an important point behind the woman's purpose. Borrowing or imposing values and purpose doesn't inspire sustainability.

The best way to inspire ourselves and others is to articulate our own purpose and allow others to do so as well. Clarity of our own purpose and where it comes from enables us to be grounded in what is important. As we draw confidence from core beliefs and purpose, rather than from other people's positioning, we are more likely to respect their purpose and values even when based on different beliefs.[19] We can work together better when we are clear about who we are as individuals.

Together, we helpers pursue a goal of making the world healthier, but each person brings their unique spin to this greater effort. Enrique, a Honduran medical student, provides a great example of this. He discovered greater purpose, direction, and motivation through writing a personal purpose statement.

"Before I was in medical school, I had a lot of anxiety," explained Enrique. "I didn't know what I was supposed to do with my life. I didn't have a clear understanding of my own values and purpose, so I was led more by other people's beliefs. After writing my core values and purpose statement, I was surprised at how much relief I felt, because now I knew how to make better decisions. My purpose statement seems like a light that traces my path toward goals, guides me as I make difficult decisions, and helps me thrive in the most difficult moments."

A purpose statement brings together core beliefs, values, virtues, strengths, motivations, and hopes. This work is focused on our own development, but it helps us engage in healthier social connections and influence. Understanding our purpose fosters the ability to be better family members, spouses, friends, team members, and community participants. This individualistic activity helps us to be collectively effective.

Voices from the Field: Apply purpose to every part of life.

"I learned I need to approach my profession as a life ministry. The sense of purpose has helped to sustain me so I can help others at traumatic times. I do a lot of switching hats, but they all cover the same bald head." Charles, Paramedic, United States

Your purpose statement does not need to inspire anyone but you. It should be memorable so you can easily recall what is important. It lifts up purposeful, intentional living for you and only you.[20] A well-written statement works for all life stages, from early adulthood through post-retirement. Because we are so much more than our career or caring role, it is important to develop one statement that applies in every context. Your purpose statement should pertain to how you live as a family member, professional, friend, and member of society at all ages.

Knowing our own purpose enables us to be grounded in what is important, make decisions based on who we feel called to be, and keep moving forward even when the journey gets hard. Savor moments when you experience your purpose making a difference in the world. Keep encouraging notes to remind yourself of such moments. Powerful purpose goes a step beyond helping others to include personal wellness.[21]

Develop Balanced Purpose for Self-Care

As a caregiver at heart, I know exactly what it's like to fall into the trap of thinking care of others is more important than care of self. Taking care of Ken as he faced the end of his life and helping others after the September 11 attacks was just one example of a time when it was too easy to put aside personal needs. At such times, I found the sneaky, destructive message "You are being selfish" creeping into desires for self-care. Helping others during dire times can make it even harder to honor the importance of our own care.

I had to counter the thought that self-care is selfish, so I included a reminder in my purpose statement to promote my own well-being. The purpose statement I developed at that difficult time still applies today: "I will glorify God and promote healthy living characterized by love, kindness, peace, honesty, and hope." The phrase "promote healthy living" reminds me self-care needs to be a part of my purpose to really help others.

Voices from the Field: See past today's challenges.

"Learning to be intentional in everything we do helps us to always walk in our purpose, and we can maintain emotional stability because our focus is on something bigger than the situation we are going through at that moment." Miriam, Nonprofit Professional, Honduras

---

A well-designed purpose statement promotes balanced, healthy living for you and the people you relate to. For example, a health-care provider could develop the purpose statement "I will bring healing into the world." This statement is easy to remember, and if it reminds her of important values, virtues, and core beliefs, then it will be helpful. For the statement to really help, it has to convey a balance of healing for self and others. In other words, the statement should be interpreted as, "I will bring healing into the world for others and myself."

Your purpose statement will have much more meaning to you than to anyone else. In fact, it really does not need to make sense to other people. If you're reminded of your core beliefs and motivators when you think of your statement, then it's doing a good job. It will provide guidance and hope at times of loss, change, and conflict. Your purpose statement will help you shine as an individual and work more effectively with others.

WRITE YOUR PURPOSE STATEMENT

Start by writing a summary of what you articulated as core to who you are. Be creative and play with words that strike you as significant. Keep it short and simple. You can make your statement more memorable by using a metaphor or acronym. For example, "I will bring HOPE into the world" could be a purpose statement with HOPE standing for Healing, Optimism, Peace, and Empowerment. Write and edit as many times as needed to arrive at a statement you feel captures who you are called to be and gives direction for your life journey.

Voices from the Field: Use your strengths to help the team.

"If everyone brings a little something to the table, it isn't long until there is a feast. Everyone has a talent that can make the team better. Find your talent and make the team better." Mark, Firefighter, United States

Help Groups Function with Unified Purpose

How do you bring people with different skills and drives together? Shared purpose. A soccer team is more successful if players work together to score goals. A rock band performs better if individual band members make sounds that blend together to create music. Each member contributes toward the group's purpose, not just to benefit their own achievement.

Shared purpose also promotes effectiveness and sustainability in teams focused on helping others.[22] This may seem like common sense, but it can be hard to overcome societal pressures to focus on individual success. The best teams work toward a shared purpose and focus on the team's success.

Here are some strategies to increase united purpose:

- Promote awareness of organizational and professional values and purpose. Communicate core values frequently and in a variety of ways, especially when making decisions.

- When hiring team members or applying for positions, make purpose and values central to the process. Individuals whose personal values and purpose align with organizational values and purpose can work more sustainably and effectively.[23]

- Discuss important values and how to live them out in daily responsibilities. Begin meetings with a conversation about how to make values and purpose a daily reality. Ask for specific examples and bring humor into the discussion so it is more memorable.

- Define team values, virtues, and purpose as a group, based on those defined by the organization. Develop a unique catchphrase or description for the group that models the organization's perspective.

- Affirm actions that reflect organizational values and purpose.

- Provide learning and social service opportunities that promote individual and team development based on a common purpose.

Together, we can help others in more ways than we ever can alone. We find inspiration in knowing we are not alone and are part of something bigger than ourselves. "Me" becomes "we" when facing challenges and striving to make the world a better place.

Bring Your Best Forward

Having clarity of values and virtues and writing a purpose statement provides the rudder that helps us travel in a desired direction even when winds are blowing different ways. This is true for individuals and groups. However, the statements we create are helpful only if they actually are used in daily living. I have seen many organizations post beautifully articulated statements on the walls, but actions reflect other influences—especially finances. Healthy functioning is more sustainable when we live in ways that align with what we believe is important.[24]

We increase resilience and counter challenges such as burnout with a balanced purpose that promotes care of self and others.[25] Now that we know how to clarify what is important, we will look at how to apply purpose and values to the journey. We will take the next step toward resilient and sustainable caring by defining our best, balanced selves along with identifying the boundaries needed to stay on track. Guided by purpose, our goodness shines brighter as it is revealed through daily expressions of care.

GUIDE TO THRIVE STRATEGIES

1. Commit to being intentional about who you are and increase self-differentiation.

2. Identify and articulate important values, virtues, and beliefs.

3. Know and use strengths and growth areas.

4. Claim and reclaim the motivations leading you to a helping role.

5. Develop a purpose statement that reminds you what is important.

6. Include self-care in how you define important values and purpose.

7. Help your family, team, or organization know and function according to their important values, virtues, and purpose.

Discussion Questions

Recall a situation when you were helping others and felt overwhelmed. What helped you?

Did articulating core beliefs and values lead to any discoveries about yourself? If so, what?

What role do virtues play in your helping work?

How do you think personal values and purpose help when helping others is hard?

What does a balanced purpose mean for you?

How can you promote purpose within groups?

Chapter 3

PROMOTE YOUR BEST, BALANCED SELF WITH HEALTHY BOUNDARIES

We establish energy reserves and radiate our goodness more easily when honoring healthy boundaries.

Foster Balance and Resilience

Being our best, balanced self takes intentional work. Pressures and threats will challenge our efforts, so we need to live in a way that enables us to reflect important values and thrive. Recently, my adult children jokingly reminisced about a less-than-ideal Karen moment.

On a warm summer day, I juggled watching our three young children and working from home. While outside playing on the swing set, one of my sons pushed a boy who had hit my other son. Later we were enjoying dinner and conversing about the day when the boy's mother called. Fatigue and maternal emotions took over my ability to reason.

"Your son attacked my son!" she said. "Your son bullied my son!" I yelled back. We both failed to listen and respond thoughtfully. The conversation ended with yelling and repeatedly slamming the phone.

I sheepishly returned to dinner facing my family's shocked expressions. Now I can laugh about that less-than-ideal reaction, but a part of me still cringes. Yes, human, but not what I want to reflect.

True, I was exhausted and struggling to find balance among family, career, family business, and community involvement. However, knowing this did not help me feel better about my response. It just pointed to my need for intentionality, boundaries, and balance. I needed to intentionally apply what was important to daily living and establish limits so I could be at my best for each piece of life.

Are you remembering any cringeworthy reactions? We all have human moments when we fall short of our ideal. The resulting guilt or embarrassment indicates we have gone astray from who we want to be. Living in ways aligned with important values, virtues, and purpose is far more sustainable than a landscape filled with regrets. Staying on the path of integrity takes continued effort due to the constant pull by emotions, pressures, and challenges.

Your best, balanced self is the healthy you radiating internal goodness. It is not the perfect you in a perfect life. If the phrase "best self" pulls you into perfectionism mode, stop! Life is a mixture of things and seldom perfect. When we are at our best, we have a healthy attitude about ourselves, others, and the world. We radiate what is important despite circumstances, and we honor boundaries to make this possible. Ideally, our best self reflects authentic living with balance in our perspectives, resources, and relationships—especially when challenged.

To live at our healthy best, we need to know what that looks like. Once we clarify how our best, balanced self looks, we can develop the boundaries and resilience needed to stay on a sustainable path. In helping roles, it is important to consider emotional responsibility and how to promote healthy limits among others. All of this is part of supporting your best, balanced self to thrive and experience the joys of a caring journey.

///

Resilience at Work: Imagine . . .

Someone has pushed your buttons. You want to yell and humiliate. You want to react in a way that expresses the frustration boiling inside. While this may seem satisfying for a moment, you know such a reaction will eat at your conscience. So instead, you take a moment to collect runaway thoughts and recall what is important.

With values, virtues, and purpose in mind, you calmly respond. Perhaps you show patience, wisdom, respect, and honesty. Whether or not there is resolution, you can close your eyes at the end of the day knowing there is nothing to be ashamed about. Your integrity is intact. Just as important, you grow more confident in the ability to respond as your best, healthiest self even when it is difficult. Yep, you can deal with tough stuff.

///

Define and Support Your Best, Balanced Self

If you created an image of your best, balanced self, what would it look like? Let's say a different color represents each important value, virtue, and purpose. The center of your image represents the healthy you adorned with an array of beautiful colors. The outer edges stand for various life roles. No matter what the landscape looks like, the central image representing the best part of you remains eye-catching. Hues may vary, but the colorful beauty of your best self remains.

Consider the different colors—the values, virtues, beliefs, and purpose that form the core of who you are. Think about how to reflect those important pieces in daily living.

- When life is good and you feel as though you are responding well to needs, what attitudes do you radiate?

- When challenged or mistreated, how can you reflect core beliefs?

- If confronted with an unexpected tragedy, what does demonstrating important virtues and beliefs look like?

- When exposed to someone else's suffering, how does your best self respond?

- At home after a tough day, how do you demonstrate top values?

- How do important virtues and purpose show in the way you treat yourself?

Although it may be difficult at times to respond in ways that reflect our best selves, doing so is more sustainable than reacting impulsively.[1] It takes intentional efforts, but the payoff includes personal wellness, integrity, resilience, and sustainability. Strengthening resilience includes seeing ourselves handle challenges with competence while being who we want to be.[2] Despite situational changes, core beliefs and purpose can provide a wonderful guide to healthy living when applied to life's journey.

> *One's philosophy is not best expressed in words; it is expressed in the choices one makes. In the long run, we shape our lives, and we shape ourselves. The process never ends until we die.* —Eleanor Roosevelt

Wherever I am working, I make sure to have a framed copy of my purpose statement centrally positioned on my desk. I also have it on my phone, computer, and desk at home. I know it by memory, but visual reminders help when something unexpected momentarily jumbles my brain. While dealing with difficult situations, I take a breath, remember my purpose statement, and thoughtfully respond rather than react in ways I may regret.

REMEMBER WHAT IS IMPORTANT AND APPLY IT TO DAILY LIFE

Make reminders of what you articulated as important, especially your purpose statement. Be creative and use various formats. As you consider values, virtues, and purpose, clarify what you look like at your best in a variety of situations. Be specific, describing thoughts, words, and actions. How do you treat others and yourself in various scenarios when being at your best?

Again, this is not the perfect self you may be tempted to define, but the balanced, happy, ethical, effective self you are striving toward. Write a description of the presence you want to bring into the world based on what you defined as important.

Think of how you would like to be remembered after dying. This sounds morbid, but it really gets us to think about choices, attitudes, and priorities. Use mental imagery to see yourself responding as you hope to.

During one memorable occasion, a staff member sat across from me in my church office while complaining, shouting, and even threatening me because of candles. I could not believe candles would upset anyone to such a degree. I was tempted to point out how overreactive and unreasonable he was being, which would have escalated an already difficult situation. Instead, I looked at my purpose statement and responded with important values in mind. A thoughtful response defused the situation and reflected who I feel called to be.

The explosive encounter shook me up, but I continued through the day with a sense of integrity. I did hold him accountable for poor behavior, but I acted with calm direction rather than impulsive anger. It was only with intentionality that I could reflect my values, especially kindness and peace, in such an emotional encounter. Processing the situation later with people outside of the organization helped me become grounded again. A great support crew who can remind and encourage us as we work to be at our best is an invaluable asset.

Striving to be our healthiest, best selves is not a solo act. Support from others gives us strength to respond with integrity during emotionally charged situations. At times, I have shared my purpose statement with a few safe people, asking them to help me remember what I am striving toward. This is a gift you can offer to others as well. Colleagues can give perspective, reminding us we are a part of something bigger than ourselves. Support crews cannot do our work, but may encourage us on the wonderful and challenging journey of helping others.

Voices from the Field: Intentionally model important values.

"I tell my staff we need to help and respect others even when they do not treat us that way. People can be jealous and judgmental, especially when you are in a leadership position. This is normal. But we don't have to be like them. It is important to model good behaviors. We can help each other do that." Sonia, Children's Home Director, Honduras

---

Relationships are vital for healthy living, but they also create pressures that pull us in different directions.[3] This is where healthy boundaries help, especially when expectations are high. Boundaries differentiate us from others, making it possible to apply personal beliefs to life. As we honor healthy boundaries, we decrease the influence of anxiety and foster resilient caring.[4]

Connect Healthy Boundaries with Sustainability

We caregivers often hear about the importance of healthy boundaries, but seldom receive adequate training to clarify what this means. A helpful example of boundaries occurred when my young sons were tasked with cleaning their bedroom. Colorful Legos, books, and Matchbox cars covered the floor. Dirty clothes strewn on the furniture created a stale odor. After slipping on a toy, I hollered, "You need to clean your room before you can do anything else."

At first, the boys yelled at each other about who had to do what. I tried to tune out the noise, hoping it wouldn't end with tears, but then was struck by the silence. I looked in the bedroom and was astonished by their ingenuity. They had created a line with tape across the floor designating who had to do what. It was magical. The boys cleaned their room while encouraging each other. The boundary clarified each person's responsibility.

We can't always use tape, but there are many times we need to know where to draw the line designating what we are and are not responsible for, what we can and should not do. Boundaries relate to physical, emotional, and cognitive limits that promote healthy balance.[5] Healthy limits go a long way in preventing secondary traumatic stress and other challenges.[6]

Some people and organizations have insatiable needs, so honoring limits can be difficult. However, personal and group sustainability relies on healthy boundaries.[7] Sarah learned this while working for a nonprofit organization that helped vulnerable families.

"People keep asking me to do more when I just want to have time with my young family. I feel exhausted, but can't say no without feeling guilty," Sarah tearfully explained. She initially thrived when the organization expanded her role. Over time, her passion turned into resentment, and she blamed others for her difficulties. Sarah abruptly resigned, creating division and anxiety in the struggling organization. Lack of healthy boundaries led to an unsustainable situation, regardless of how talented or admirable Sarah's work was.

Voices from the Field: Be intentional about roles and boundaries.

"When you live in a small community, as a professional it can be really hard to know what boundaries are healthy. Many people want you to be a friend, and you are expected to be a part of the community, but there are leadership expectations that can be very different. It's also hard because people communicate now in so many different ways and expect immediate responses. Figuring out boundaries is hard but important work." Scott, Pastor, United States

When we don't understand boundaries or see them as a negative like Sarah did, then it is difficult to set them for ourselves and respect other people's boundaries. Healthy boundaries not only help us care for others more sustainably, but help the people and organizations we work with function more effectively.[8] When we assume responsibility for more than we can handle, we risk burnout and diminish opportunities for others. Worse yet, a lack of boundaries can lead to unethical or unsafe situations.

I know how important boundaries are for safety. Early in my career, Ned, the head of staff, made comments about my appearance and caressed my hand. I experienced firsthand the negatives caused by a lack of boundaries, and I made sure I was never alone with him again. About a year later, Ned was fired due to inappropriate behaviors with multiple women. This experience emphasized a valuable lesson: pay attention to internal alarms, as they most likely indicate a breach of important boundaries.

Social pressures can make it difficult to understand or respond even when internal alarms are sounding. There's seldom a clear indication when a line between right and wrong has been crossed.[9] General lack of understanding about limits leads to fuzzy or nonexistent boundaries. In helping roles, emotional boundaries are among the most difficult to clarify and honor.[10]

Know Your Emotional Responsibility

Think about an emotionally intense time when you helped someone:

- What was your role?
- What emotions did the other person express?
- What was your emotional response before, during, and after?
- What was your emotional responsibility in the difficult moment?
- What are fair expectations regarding the emotions you carried forward?

Emotional boundaries identify what we are emotionally responsible for. Put simply: my emotions are mine, and your emotions are yours. You are not responsible for assuming my emotions, nor should I take on yours. This is true for people we don't know and those we are very close to. Emotional boundaries help us discern where our own emotions end and another person's emotions begin. We are going to be influenced by the people we help, but we do not need to, nor should we, take on their emotions and suffering.[11]

Voices from the Field: Increase the ability to regulate emotions.

"I learned early in my career that I needed to be able to show I care, but I also needed to be able to flip a switch. It was common to have an appointment where I had to share a cancer diagnosis, immediately followed by a healthy puppy exam. The puppy's owners didn't know what I had to deal with earlier, nor should they have. In order to give each client my best, I have to be fully present and able to move on to the next. Another reality is I want to go home and enjoy my family without carrying all of the day's emotions." Steve, Veterinarian, United States

Consideration of emotional responsibility leads us to look at empathy, a highly promoted virtue in helping professions. "Empathy," in its original Greek, literally means feeling what others feel.[12] Empathy has a role, but we need to keep it in perspective. Our emotions can be tiring enough without adding those of others.[13] As James, a physician, said, "How are we supposed to feel what our patients are feeling when we can't know exactly what they're experiencing? Also, I can't imagine having the energy to take on every patient's emotion."

Empathy fosters compassion by helping us connect to another's experience.[14] However, we shouldn't try to assume their emotional journey.[15] Compassion includes awareness of suffering accompanied by a desire to alleviate that suffering.[16] It honors emotional boundaries, allowing people to experience their own journey.[17] When we confuse compassion with empathy, we give up emotional distinctiveness and risk our work becoming more about our own needs.

Compassion fatigue really could be understood as fatigue from empathy.[18] A balance of compassion for others and ourselves replenishes the energy empathy demands. Self-compassion expands the ability to experience our own emotions while being in the midst of others' emotions and trauma. We can be compassionate and experience our own life journeys.[19]

Emotional boundaries allow us to help people without their journeys rattling ours too much.[20] Differentiating between ourselves and others emotionally helps us take responsibility for our own emotions without trying to do so for others.[21] Self-awareness is key to recognizing the influence of other people's emotions and letting go of them when they weigh on us.[22] Emotional boundaries promote compassion while also allowing us to experience the joy, hope, sorrow, challenges, and blessings of our own journey.[23]

USE METAPHORS TO FOSTER HEALTHY BOUNDARIES

- **Emotional Bubbles**: In anxious situations, imagine that each person involved, including you, has an emotional bubble. As you start to sense another person's anxiety, think "I am (name). I care, but I don't need to take on your emotions." Take a moment to mindfully acknowledge your own emotions and differentiate from the emotional experiences of others.[24]

- **Fenced in Yard**: Let's say each person has their own yard to maintain with a fence that designates boundaries. Your yard includes everything you are responsible for, including emotions, happiness, duties, and responses. Be creative and playful as you name what belongs in your yard. Perhaps there is a garden of joy, herbs of learning, a fountain of hope, a tree of wisdom, and even a few weeds designating pesky intrusions.

Your yard is surrounded by the yards of people in your life. Each family member, colleague, friend, and person you help has their own yard. You can support each other, but remember each person is ultimately responsible for their yard. Note what you tend to take care of in other people's yards, or expect other people to take care of in your yard, to determine where you need to establish healthy boundaries and change behaviors.

Establish Healthy Boundaries

We can promote balance with boundaries even though doing so may not come easily.[25] Katie, a hospice professional, struggled to find balance between her young family and work. She knew both were important, but found herself repeatedly agreeing to work extra shifts and missing her son's soccer games. Katie usually accepted extra work with a positive attitude, but was pressured to take six extra shifts last month. Feelings of helplessness and resentment grew as she missed family events.

Katie's contract doesn't require picking up extra shifts, but she wanted to be a good team member. She was also afraid refusal would cause negative consequences. Katie could continue picking up extra shifts whenever asked and let resentment grow. However, she loves her job, so she decided to work on setting new limits. Ideally, we start a position with healthy boundaries, but often discover we haven't maintained them. Setting new boundaries in a familiar role can be tricky, but we can promote success with the following strategies:

1. **Define boundaries based on what is important for being your best, balanced self.**

   Review the values, virtues, beliefs, and purpose you identified as important, as well as the description of your best, balanced self. This will help you approach boundaries from core beliefs, rather than emotions and relationship pressures. Boundaries aligned with what is important are much easier to honor.

2. **Identify what creates imbalance and promotes balance.**

   Imbalance usually indicates a need for healthy boundaries, so consider what makes life feel lopsided. You have already thought about what you look like at your best, balanced self; now think about when you aren't at your best. Identify when you feel a lack of balance and what you can do to regain balance. What boundaries can create harmony?

3. **Use resources.**

   Job descriptions, professional codes, and defined organizational expectations can help you make informed decisions and may hold more weight with people you are accountable to. Outside resources also can provide greater perspective.

4. **Write needed boundaries.**

   Keep boundaries simple and practical so you can honor them. Write, rewrite, and write again. Share what you develop with trusted people who can provide an objective perspective and support.[26]

5. **Identify how boundaries are mutually beneficial.**[27]

   Clarify your need for boundaries and how they will help others too. Relationship and professional sustainability are important benefits. Awareness of how boundaries promote group sustainability and effectiveness helps us find the courage to honor them.

6. **Communicate limits clearly and non-anxiously.**[28]

   Explain limits when everyone is calm. Keep it simple and be creative. For example, Faris, a physician, used a hat metaphor while working in a small town. If someone approached him with a medical question during family time, he responded, "Right now, I'm wearing my dad hat. You can call my office on Monday when I'm wearing my doctor hat."

7. **Be persistent.**

   Be prepared for resistance, because organizations and individuals will challenge limits even if those limits promote group sustainability.[29] Listen to how others are feeling and acknowledge their concerns.[30] This doesn't mean you agree with them, but that you do care. Someone else's difficulty with a limit doesn't mean you should drop it. Explain the limit in a variety of ways as many times as needed.

8. **Determine what you will and won't bend on.**

   The flexibility to handle unexpected events is important for resilience, but it is helpful to know what exceptions to allow; otherwise, it's too easy to drop boundaries for everything.[31] Know where you need to draw the line and take a stand, and then empower yourself with the courage to do so. Identify consequences and apply them calmly when others fail to honor boundaries .[32]

Let's look at how Katie applied these strategies to develop new boundaries in her hospice work. Katie knew it was important to pick up extra shifts, but she also decided some family events took priority. She noticed that more than three extra shifts each month led to her feeling imbalanced. Fatigue negatively affected her family life and her ability to deal with challenges at work. Just as important, Katie knew she was not living her best, balanced self and reflecting important values.

After reviewing important values and her job description, Katie established a new time boundary. She decided to pick up three extra shifts each month if there weren't conflicting family events. Katie knew this would positively impact team relationships and increase overall effectiveness. The new boundary helped her find the courage to say no and talk with her supervisor when needed. As we work to be at our best, balanced self and promote healthy boundaries, we model the importance of doing so to our family, team, and organization.[32]

Voices from the Field: Be present.

"I put my heart and soul into caring for people, but when I go home, I go home. We need to be fully present where we are and always be kind. When frustrated or having a long day, step back, take a breath, and be kind. We can bring our best to the people around us." Gerri, Healthcare Technician and Family Caregiver, United States

Develop Balance and Boundaries in Teams

We each have a role in influencing the balance and health of our groups. Sled dog teams provide a great example of how members affect each other. I enjoy watching teams and mushers start the three-hundred-mile John Beargrease Sled Dog Marathon. Excited barking pierces cold winter air as teams prepare to race. Each dog's harness is attached to a main lead, with six pairs extending in front of a sled. Dogs eagerly jump forward as they take off.

Twelve dogs start running with disciplined focus on completing the journey through snow-covered trails in pine forests. They are smooth and synchronized, needing only occasional directions from the musher. Each dog has a role, and all are connected. Imagine if a dog sat down or a back dog tried to take over lead dog responsibilities. Resulting imbalance and chaos would create an unsustainable journey, reducing chances of success. Boundaries and balance promote a team's optimal performance.

We may not be harnessed to other members of our teams or

families, but each person influences group functioning. Wherever we are positioned in the team, we can promote balance and effectiveness with boundaries.[33]

TIPS FOR PROMOTING BALANCE AND BOUNDARIES WITH FAMILIES OR TEAMS

- Know the presence you bring influences others positively or negatively. Respect others' boundaries and show appreciation for healthy respect of your boundaries.

- Consider how you can help your team function effectively with balance.

- Remember healthy boundaries are not one-sided—they also promote group well-being.

- Model positive ways to communicate important limits.

- Keep in mind: organizations that promote healthy boundaries show care and increase overall effectiveness.

- Create boundaries informed by organizational or team values and purpose.

- Promote group sustainability with policies and procedures based on healthy boundaries.

Be ready for resistance when establishing new boundaries. Change is difficult for any group, even though it leads to healthier functioning. Be patient and realistic. We can help others promote balanced functioning and healthier boundaries with clear, persistent communication.[34]

Our ability to establish and communicate healthy boundaries will positively affect any group we are part of. We can care wholeheartedly while experiencing our own life journey.

Increase Hope with Sustainability

There is no doubt about it—we are affected by others, especially people we care about. As we live our values and maintain healthy boundaries, we have more say in how the mix of emotions and anxieties shapes our journey. Increasing resilience and sustainability is an ongoing process. We may have leaps forward and steps back in promoting our best, balanced self. As Madeleine L'Engle wrote, "A self is not something static, tied up in a pretty parcel and handed to the child, finished and complete. A self is always becoming."[35]

Life changes needed for well-being often include boundaries to clarify what we are responsible for and what we can let go of. Positive limits help us thrive while walking in connection with others. We allow ourselves to experience our own emotional journey and allow others to do the same. As you promote your best, balanced self with helpful boundaries, you create a resilient and sustainable caring path.

All helping journeys become more sustainable with compassion for self and others. Now that we have looked at supporting our best, balanced self with healthy boundaries, we turn to self-compassion. Fostering compassion for self and others helps us honor important limits and promotes healing in the wake of broken boundaries. Self-compassion is another piece of resilience that takes intentional efforts. The journey of helping others becomes more radiant when we personally experience the transformative power of being loved and cared for.

GUIDE TO THRIVE STRATEGIES

1. Provide creative ways to remember your purpose statement, values, and virtues.

2. Establish a support crew of safe people who can remind and support you in reflecting your balanced purpose.

3. Define what your best, healthiest self looks like in a variety of situations. Use mental imagery to imagine yourself responding as you hope to.

4. Choose an image and statement to help remember that you don't need to take on other people's emotions and anxieties.

5. Discern where you need to develop healthy boundaries, articulate those boundaries for yourself, and then communicate as needed.

6. Review job descriptions and relevant professional boundaries as resources.

7. Process past and present difficult scenarios with an objective, safe person to help discern and maintain healthy boundaries.

8. Foster balance and healthy boundaries in groups.

Discussion Questions

What was it like thinking about your best, balanced self?

What thoughts do you have about boundaries, especially emotional boundaries?

Describe a situation in which you saw a lack of healthy boundaries. (Be general and don't use specific details, especially names.)

How did the lack of boundaries affect others?

Describe a setting or situation in which you saw healthy boundaries at work. (Be general and don't use specific details, especially names.)

How did the healthy boundaries affect others?

What can help you promote your best, balanced self with healthy boundaries?

How can you help others understand the importance of boundaries?

Chapter 4

FOSTER SELF-COMPASSION

We create emotional space to thrive with self-compassion.

Change the World with Compassion

Compassion changes lives. This was certainly true for Augie, a dog in a Middle Eastern country. He had been beaten, shot, and left to die in a garbage pit. There was little hope for Augie, but he captured the attention and heart of a woman walking by. Upon seeing her, Augie moved the only thing he could and wagged his tail. The woman brought him home and went to great lengths to help Augie. She sent this dog with an undefeatable spirit to the United States, where he received medical care and a loving home.

The chain of compassion that saved Augie inspired many others, including Steve, the veterinarian who provided care. He explained, "I was inspired by the person who started the process to save Augie. My role was one piece of many. I was also inspired by Augie's ability to look beyond suffering. When lying at the dump, he wagged his tail simply because he was happy to see the woman. She could easily have ignored him, but she didn't."

Augie has a home and is wagging his tail happily to greet others due to the kindness of many people. Those inspired by an act of compassion gave with generosity and kindness to continue the compassion. They positively influenced the world with care and found nourishment for their own journey. Compassion is contagious and powerful, especially when we understand its reach includes our own suffering.

We often find it easy to respond compassionately to the suffering of other people and animals, yet how likely are we to offer the same to ourselves? As talked about previously, there's a simple reality we often neglect: as we help others, we also need to care for ourselves. As Daisy, a Honduran physician, said, "We are taught a lot of different ways to help others, but not how to help ourselves." Because this rings true for many of us, we need to be intentional about fostering compassion toward ourselves.

Self-compassion generates nourishment and healing for the journey. We will take a look at compassion's role in fostering self-care and creating deeper connections. For many of us, this includes shaking off the yoke of perfectionism to promote vibrant caregiving beyond mistakes. Once we know how to foster self-compassion in our own lives, we can help others do so as well. Compassion increases resilience, makes the journey more sustainable, and fills our surroundings with beauty.

//

Resilience at Work: Imagine . . .

You offer healing and kindness amid suffering. There is a critical moment, one of those life- shifting occasions for people needing help. Despite the heart, skill, and effort you give, all does not go as hoped. A tear drops for the suffering, while that small, yet powerful voice whispers, "What if . . ." and expands the sorrow. You offer yourself a hug and kind words, and you use resources to open up a space for healing and growth. With care and strength, you stay on course. Suffering has touched your life but does not have the final word.

//

Experience Compassion's Mutual Gifts

Compassion is core to the mix of caring for others and self, because it moves us from identifying suffering toward alleviating that suffering. Often when we offer compassion to others, we experience it as well. I have experienced compassion's mutual blessing many times over the years, and one special occasion occurred while visiting Paul before he died.

"Pastor Karen, God loves you so much," said Paul as he lay in the hospital bed next to machines blinking and beeping. I was focused on providing him care, yet his words filled me up. In the midst of sadness, I felt as though a divine message was conveyed through this kind man. Paul's gift given years ago still makes my heart smile.

Think of times when you gave compassion, and someone's response touched you deeply. Remember such moments as nourishment for continued caring. Compassion comes within the blessing of connection and emphasizes our common humanity.[1] Compassion helps care speak louder than the world's brokenness. Even when we cannot change an outcome, compassion counters the loneliness and despair that accompany suffering.[2]

Voices from the Field: Find meaning with compassion.

"We can be there for people and animals. Recently, I helped an eighty-five-year-old man and his beloved dog who was at the end of life. The man was alone, so I just stayed and listened to his stories. This felt really rewarding. It is meaningful to share some part of a person's life that is tough. In being there for them, we make it easier." Lucy, Veterinarian, United States

---

Acts of compassion bring healing into our own lives as well as the people we help. The Dalai Lama explained, "The more time you spend thinking about yourself, the more suffering you will experience. The incredible thing is that when we think of alleviating other people's suffering, our own suffering is reduced."[3]

Acts of kindness toward others move us beyond focus on self to participate in something bigger than ourselves.[4] This awakens a joy and gratitude within that reaches beyond life's circumstances.[5] Emotionally intense situations can provide some of the deepest, most meaningful experiences when we can see more than suffering.

One memorable experience occurred while I walked with my mother-in-law, Ruth. Her mind was gripped by dementia, and she knew something was wrong. We slowly walked hand in hand around the garden of her new home at a care center. Birds sang and yellow flowers dotted the path, yet a heavy sadness filled the air. We occasionally stopped to cry and hug, then resumed walking while humming favorite hymns. I was struck with a grand mix of sorrow, helplessness, compassion, and love.

I could not take away Ruth's pain, but I could affirm that she mattered and make her suffering less lonely. I was blessed to be in that space with her even though it was truly sad. I may very well be on a similar journey someday, and if so, I hope I am not walking alone. Sometimes our caring presence is the best and only gift we can give.

Such simple acts that communicate "I care" provide seeds of hope amid suffering's sorrow. Together we are human, and together we can find courage to face suffering. We may even find glimpses of hope, peace, and joy amid the difficulties. A change of perception from "I am the helper and you need help" to a connection based on shared humanity leads to deeper, more meaningful ways of functioning in the midst of suffering.[6]

Voices from the Field: See the blessings.

"It was a great blessing to help my grandmother by providing the same care she had given to others over her lifetime. It was hard to see her struggle, but the blessings were much greater." Hilary, Family Caregiver and Educator, Kenya and United States

Counter Misconceptions about Self-Compassion

Self-compassion includes acknowledgment of our own humanity and suffering, followed by a kind response.[7] We honor that we, like everyone else, deserve compassion.[8] Despite this truth, we often:

- Expect too much from ourselves without offering kindness and forgiveness.

- Get stuck thinking that if we had acted differently, the outcome would have been different.

- Become caught up in and stressed out by unrealistic expectations.

- Accuse ourselves of not being tough enough.

- Think kindness will make us lazy or less proficient.

- Believe taking care of ourselves is selfish.

- Become afraid self-compassion will lead to getting stuck in self-pity.

False perceptions of self-compassion lead us away from sustainable caring. Self-compassion is a needed ally, because even when we know compassion's goodness, it is difficult to fully escape suffering's sorrow. The world's grief can strike at our hearts. Self-compassion equips us to process our own pain and move forward in hopeful ways.[9]

Harsh perceptions about self-compassion are false and destructive.[10] They break us down, create a sense that "we don't matter," and build barriers to healing. Acts of self-kindness help us become less absorbed in ourselves so we can care for others in healthier ways and learn from mistakes.[11]

Self-compassion gives us perspective to see personal struggles in the larger context of human suffering.[12] This is far more likely to increase our motivation than harsh criticism is. A healthy blend of compassion for others and self will foster our ability to see ourselves kindly and embrace hope.

Increase Vitality with Self-Compassion

What do you see when looking in a mirror? Perhaps you see the color of your hair, skin, and eyes. Maybe you notice creases marking years of stress and smiles. As you look deeper, you see the hopes, dreams, beauty, and imperfections peeking out from your gaze.

Whatever we see, there is something we cannot deny—we are human. Self-compassion involves acknowledging our own human suffering with a nonjudgmental awareness.[13] We can foster this with four components:

1. Recognize our common humanity and shake off perfectionism.
2. Notice personal suffering.
3. Be kind to ourselves.
4. Offer self-forgiveness.[14]

Simple acts of self-compassion enable us to remain connected with ourselves and others in healthy ways.

1. Recognize Our Common Humanity and Shake Off Perfectionism.

I had asked a group of family practice residents to each write down a recurring fear or negative thought they struggled with. "I don't know enough," wrote one of the medical residents during this self-compassion activity. Each resident passed their statement to a partner, who read it as if it was their own fear. The actual owner of the thought then provided encouragement.

Participants easily supported a colleague when they would have been inclined to treat themselves harshly. As I listened to activity partners converse, I noticed all eight participants unknowingly had written down the same thought. When I pointed this out, there was a collective breath. Knowing they shared a common struggle empowered the residents.

I described this "aha" moment to experienced physicians, who all said: "I still struggle with feeling like I don't know enough!" It doesn't matter how smart or experienced we are: helping others will be hard and will remind us of our limitations. Despite the challenges, we can find comfort in knowing we don't struggle alone.

Self-compassion recognizes that we, like all other humans, are fallible, experience difficult feelings, and respond positively to kindness.[15] When we shift self-perception to include similarities with others, we are able to move away from hurtful comparisons and judgments. Authentic, sustainable compassion is grounded in our hopes to alleviate suffering along with awareness of our own humanity. Being human implies many things, including imperfection.

Perfectionism runs deep within my DNA, so I have spent a significant amount of time and energy loosening its harsh grip on my life. I know too well its oppressive partners, such as comparison, judgment, and shame. Shame is particularly dangerous, as it messes with our longing for connection with others.[16] Shame is not about something we did, but about who we are. Shame screams falsehoods, claiming, "You are not worthy."

Contrary to that message, each one of us is worthy of being accepted, affirmed, and loved. Let me repeat this important message— you are worthy of being accepted, cared for, and loved. Even with all of your imperfections. Shame denies this, of course, and promotes isolation by creating a false need to hide what we perceive as lacking or wrong.[17] Embrace your humanity to shake off the unfair, even cruel expectations of perfectionism.

Voices from the field: Don't step on the pedestal.

"Society wants its professionals to be perfect. It's easy to start believing we can or should be. You get put on a pedestal, and it's hard to live up to those expectations, because we are all human. We have to resist such projections and not step onto the pedestal. We all disappoint people at times and make mistakes. Communicate to yourself and others, 'I will do my humanly best, but sometimes that's not enough.'" Faris, Physician, United States

---

Our humanity limits what we can do. Even with all the technology in the world, we won't be able to fix or save all the people and animals we help. We need to try, yes, but we also are required to accept the limitations inherent in reality. This does not nullify the power of compassion. We can see the beauty in genuine acts of compassion, even amid tragedy, with a perceptual shift that acknowledges unrealistic expectations.[18]

FACE UNREALISTIC EXPECTATIONS

- List unfair expectations you struggle with. Differentiate between high functioning and perfection. Write a separate list of expectations that are reasonable and within your control. Acknowledge unreasonable expectations for what they are: unrealistic, unfair, and unhelpful.
- Talk with trusted colleagues, mentors, mental health-care providers, and safe people for additional perspective.
- Give yourself permission to be human. Symbolically let go of unfair expectations by writing them down, and then crumpling and throwing away the paper. Personalize and recite part of the Serenity Prayer by Reinhold Niebuhr:[19]

  God, give me the grace to
  accept with serenity the things that cannot be changed,
  courage to change the things that should be changed,
  and the wisdom to distinguish the one from the other.

Together, we bring hope based on our human giftedness and limitations. Resist the temptation to set yourself apart with perfectionism. Allow yourself to be wonderfully human. Love and care for yourself in the midst of vulnerabilities and imperfections.[20] Counter shame with honest sharing.[21] We will consider this important task further in chapter 8's section *Overcome Silencers.* Self-compassion helps us walk on a collective path, not as outsiders but as people who also need care.

Voices from the Field: Allow yourself to be human.

"I am a perfectionist, and this can make it really hard to be sustainable. Perfectionism makes it easy to beat up on yourself. Learn to be good to yourself. Learn from mistakes, but don't dwell on them, and remember the good you are doing." Mike, Veterinarian, United States

---

2. Notice Personal Suffering.

As part of the human tapestry, we are more likely to respond compassionately to our suffering when we are mindful of its presence. Let's take a look in the metaphorical mirror again. Look past the color of your hair and the shape of your nose to see the experiences etched on your mind and heart. What experiences and emotions stand out? Self-compassion urges us to notice the great variety of life, including the reality of our own suffering.

Mindful awareness promotes acceptance of the present moment without labeling it good or bad.[22] This practice increases the ability to regulate emotions and decrease anxiety, so we will also look at it in chapter 5. Mindfulness moves us to recognize feelings as an ever-changing part of our human experience. Learning to sit with our own emotions helps us be with other people in the midst of their emotions, especially when we remain differentiated.

Regular awareness of personal suffering decreases the interference

of pain while we work with other people's suffering. We can acknowledge difficult emotions and process them at a time when it is safe to do
so. A daily routine with even a few minutes committed to mindfulness
is helpful. Meditation, prayer, and just being silent while walking in
nature are wonderful ways to be thoughtful about well-being. Key to
mindfulness is calmly noting emotions, physical sensations, and other
experiences in that moment.

CREATE MINDFUL MOMENTS

- Sit comfortably, focus on breathing, and allow yourself to
  be still. Note how you are feeling physically and emotionally
  without judging it as good or bad.[23] Don't try to change
  or solve anything, but allow yourself to accept the present
  moment as it is. Acknowledge how you are doing without
  fear or judgment.
- Take a deep breath regularly throughout the day and note
  how you are feeling without judging or fixing it. At times of
  struggle, end the moment with a hug and kind words.
- Begin quiet activities such as prayers, meditation, and yoga
  with a moment of mindfulness.
- Try a guided compassion meditation.

Changing emotions are a reality we all experience.[24] Feelings have
a powerful presence in the journey of caring for others, but we can
walk the journey with more than emotions guiding us.[25] Purpose
and values provide more sustainable motivation for how we live than
fluctuating emotions. As we ground our work of helping others in

important values and purpose, we function more holistically and include our head, heart, and soul.

A healthy combination of reason, emotions, and faith is a powerful mix for promoting resilience and sustainability. Together, they help us face the difficult with strength, purpose, and hope. As important as it is, practicing mindfulness does not come naturally in our busy, noisy world.[26] Many distractions demand our attention, so we need to be intentional about creating moments of calm. Even the briefest moments open up space to offer ourselves kindness.

3. Be Kind to Ourselves.

Self-kindness includes honest, caring introspection rather than jumping to judgment. A group of fluffy gray kittens reminded Louise of this. The kittens wiggled and pounced as she examined them. After years of veterinary experience, she expected this to be a typical wellness check of healthy kittens as she treated them for ear mites.

Minutes later, one kitten was breathing heavily, and then another also went into respiratory distress. Louise and her team flew into action to save the kittens, which did recover. She explained, "When I first practiced, I would have negatively judged myself right away. After years of experience, I can respond in a kinder way that helps me process what happened. The kittens' reaction most likely happened because of unknown preexisting causes. Now I can open myself up to such possibilities, and that is a nice thing."

True compassion is inclusive. It works to alleviate the suffering of others and ourselves. We defy the harshness of perfectionism and the brokenness of the world when we offer kindness to ourselves. Self-care counters unrealistic expectations and fears that make it harder to face challenges. As we respond compassionately to ourselves, we move past self-criticisms and fears to live from a deeper sense of purpose.[27]

Purpose-driven motivation nurtured by kindness is more sustainable than fear-driven motivation. When we remove fear as a primary force, we spend less energy protecting our self-esteem and allow more room for learning, creativity, and important values.[28] We are driven by what we find most fulfilling, instead of by self-doubts, anxieties, and criticisms.

Making self-compassion real in practical ways is as simple as noticing how we treat and talk to ourselves. When you struggle or fall short of expectations, what first runs through your mind? If your automatic responses are different from what you would say to someone else, think about why. Remember, your values, virtues, and purpose should apply to the way you treat both yourself and others. Noticing our internal narrative is one way to examine how we take care of ourselves.

A negative narrative decreases resilience as hurtful thoughts attack the confidence and creativity you need to deal with challenges.[29] You know the messages. They go something like this: "You're stupid"; "You don't know enough"; or "What a weakling . . ." These internal messages based on negative and incomplete perceptions often are all too familiar.

The "not enough" notion is dominant in many societies and organizations, so it's not surprising if we internalize it. An important step in being kind to ourselves is changing such negative self-talk.[30] Standing up to our inner critic by strengthening our inner caregiver is an important way to build resilience. Recognize recurrent negative messages and change them to more positive, honest messages. Even when we know negative internal messages aren't true, they're still destructive.

COUNTER NEGATIVE SELF-TALK

Identify negative statements that tend to jump into your thinking, and then develop more supportive responses. For example, if "You're so stupid" breaks into your thinking, change the response to something like "Yep, I made a mistake, but I can deal with this." A kinder response is far less damaging and more honest, and it encourages you to deal with challenges in healthy ways. Supplement positive self-talk with a hug to yourself.

Self-kindness and positive thinking help us see better the goodness in our lives and remind us of our connection to the rest of humanity. We promote resilience when we are part of our support crew rather than our harshest judge. Sometimes, the ultimate act of kindness we can offer to ourselves is forgiveness.

> *Our human compassion binds us the one to the other—not in pity or patronizingly, but as human beings who have learnt how to turn our common suffering into hope for the future.* —Nelson Mandela

4. Offer Self-Forgiveness.

"You need to offer yourself forgiveness every night" was the sage advice given by an experienced physician after being asked what helps him deal with mistakes. Offering genuine kindness and compassion to ourselves includes the forgiveness that promotes healing and growth.

Mercy provides the stepping stones to move on from mistakes, whether they have been slight missteps or giant leaps from our path.

Forgiveness is not the easiest path to take, but it is the most sustainable one for a long journey. When we fail to forgive, we shackle ourselves to the past and the pain, making it difficult to move forward.[31] We break the shackles and recognize our humanity when we choose to forgive. Forgiveness moves us to let go of pain, judgment, and bitterness to embrace peace and healing.

Mercy allows a way filled with new possibilities. This does not mean we forget or accept a wrong as being right. Forgiveness does not condone injustice or irresponsibility. It does require us to face obligations, confront consequences, and seek to make amends. Mercy toward ourselves enables the honest learning needed to prevent repeating mistakes.[32] Self-forgiveness allows us to let go of cycles of self-directed punishment and peacefully move forward.

PRACTICE SELF-FORGIVENESS

- Face yourself in the mirror and say what you need to forgive. Look yourself in the eye and say, "I forgive you." A verbal gift of forgiveness does not take the place of making amends but accompanies such efforts.[33] If you have faith in a higher being, include awareness of divine mercy, saying, "God forgives you, and so do I." Keep repeating as long as you experience the heaviness of guilt.

- Live like someone who is forgiven. Healing happens when we go through the motions.[34]

- Talk with safe people, including professional helpers, for encouragement and perspective.

- Develop creative rituals to symbolize letting go of guilt and embracing forgiveness. Do something simple, like tossing a stone into a lake or planting a tree.

- Offer acts of kindness and generosity to express joy in moments of healing.

- Learn about the concept of divine grace. God's grace is the unconditional love and forgiveness that provides hope and healing like nothing else.

No one step or misstep defines who we are. Forgiveness helps us find grace-filled moments to fuel our journey forward.[35] We can thrive in the wide spectrum of what it means to be human. Gifted, imperfect, driven, and limited. Learn from the wisdom of others who have made mistakes yet continued to experience the beauty of helping others.

Voices from the Field: Wisdom on dealing with mistakes

"Know that no one is perfect. I'm not perfect, and you're not perfect. Learn from mistakes and be compassionate toward yourself. We need to accept vulnerability so we can help ourselves." Marlon, Dentist, Honduras

"How we respond to mistakes is key. There is strength in humility and taking responsibility, and it helps us move forward." Lisa, Firefighter, United States

"You will make mistakes. Everybody does. Apologize, then pick one or two lessons you and others can learn from the mistake. Often times, mistakes involve many people at different levels within an organization. Processing them in an honest, non-blaming way offers invaluable insights and helps the whole organization." Collins, Nurse, United States and Kenya

"We need to have forgiveness for ourselves and others so we can learn from mistakes and not repeat them. Process mistakes with others so they can promote growth and proficiency." Allen, Firefighter, United States and International

"Don't tie your identity to mistakes. Don't go into 'I made a mistake, so I can't be a good veterinarian.' Acknowledge real life, where you can't control everything and you are human." Lauren, Veterinarian, United States

"Look back, but don't stare. We need to consider if there was something we did that affected outcomes, learn, and move on to continue helping others." Wade, Physician, United States

"Everybody can make a mistake, so see yourself as a human being who is not perfect. Think about what you can learn and how to become better. When we can do this with colleagues, we can learn a lot and support each other." Irene, Nurse, Australia and Kenya

---

Foster Compassionate Families and Teams

Our actions can speak louder than what we say. Kevin, an ambulance EMT, observed, "We are told many times in training that when we are going to an emergency, it's not our emergency. If we make it our emergency, then we shouldn't be there. A calm leader promotes a more effective team and helps patients. I have learned more about why this is important and how to remain calm by observing experienced EMTs."

Each time we model a behavior, including self-compassion, we provide a learning experience. We encourage others to practice a healthy blend of compassion for themself and other people when we make it a reality in our own lives. Empowering the balance of self-compassion and compassion for others is a win-win for teams.

Balanced compassion fosters growth and effectiveness, because people are less likely to get stuck in challenges.[36] The fear of failure is replaced with a mindset geared toward group success. Our teams are infused with a "You are valued, and you can do this!" attitude.

Voices from the Field: We need to create healthier cultures.

"The prevailing culture used to be that we can't make mistakes, so we couldn't talk about them. This produced a lot of fear. We need to understand that mistakes happen. A strong team knows this and doesn't get into blaming or shaming. High-stakes mistakes almost always happen because of multiple system factors, so we need to develop an atmosphere where we can talk about mistakes to prevent future ones." Laurie, Nurse, United States

---

STRATEGIES TO PROMOTE COMPASSION IN GROUPS

- Use opportune moments for authentic sharing. Experienced team members are especially valuable in helping younger colleagues understand the need for and possibility of self-compassion when dealing with challenges.

- Model self-compassion after making a mistake.

- Promote use of resources to deal with mistakes and tragic outcomes, such as group processing and mental health-care providers.

- Help teams thrive by influencing policies and procedures to reflect an atmosphere that recognizes the importance of kindness and openness.

- Offer educational opportunities for concepts such as compassion.

- Make sure responses to mistakes reflect care for everyone involved. This does not negate accountability—but it promotes integrity and creates a just environment.

- Create a balanced mission statement and values to reflect care of employees as well as people the organization serves.

We can help create an environment that promotes resilient and sustainable caring with daily expressions of compassion, especially when people are struggling. Teams and organizations based on a culture of care are far more likely to inspire people than those based on shame.

Journey Toward a More Compassionate, Less Anxious World

The more we foster compassion for ourselves, the more we can influence others to do so. In the process, we become intimately aware of our connections and increase a capacity for resilience and growth.[37] Through compassion, we find the strength and courage to wade with hope into even the darkest places.

We often find it easy to offer compassion to others but also need to provide it intentionally to ourselves. We do this by honoring our humanity with mindful awareness of our own suffering, and then responding with kindness. Self-forgiveness is an important piece, helping us let go of the pain associated with limitations and mistakes. Like every other human being we encounter, we long for and deserve compassion. Let's make self-compassion as contagious as compassion and paint the world with hope.

Self-compassion promotes the ability to walk in the midst of challenges while honoring our own experiences. The powerful combination of self-compassion, purpose, and boundaries gives us a jump on making the journey less stressful. Now we will take the next step to decrease anxiety even more. Simple perceptual shifts change how we experience the pressures pulling us in different directions. Our responses determine whether the journey is easier or harder, kinder or harsher, stressful or peaceful.

Ready to make your journey more peaceful? Let's go!

GUIDE TO THRIVE STRATEGIES

1. Promote compassion and kindness to others and self.

2. See the positives and meaning behind compassionate acts, despite the brokenness.

3. Let go of unrealistic expectations and shame.

4. Replace negative internal narratives with more truthful, positive narratives.

5. Develop ways to share your story and vulnerabilities with safe people.

6. Increase awareness of your shared connection with humanity.

7. Practice mindfulness.

8. Meditate or pray with a focus on compassion. A guided meditation is included in the introspective activities. You also can find a wonderful array of guided meditations online.

9. Foster forgiveness toward yourself.

10. Encourage self-compassion among others.

Discussion Questions

What ideas from the chapter stand out to you?

What connection is there between compassion for others and compassion for self?

Why may we find it hard to be compassionate toward ourselves?

How can you promote self-compassion on a daily basis?

How can you foster compassion and self-compassion in your family or team?

Do you have any other thoughts regarding compassion?

Chapter 5

Decrease Anxiety

We expand resilience by moving forward based on what's important, rather than being pushed around by anxiety.

Return to Calm

Anxiety can move us in many directions. It certainly was a motivating force as I ran down the hill, afraid for my life, with twenty-five cows thundering after me. Steve and I were at his parents' farm, walking across the sunny field spotted with clover. Suddenly the cattle started running, and I jumped to life with the herd in pursuit.

My heart was racing and legs pumping as I glanced behind to see Steve laughing. I realized it wasn't a dangerous stampede bearing down, but a group of cows excited to move to the next pasture. My city-girl panic response was to ignore Steve and keep running, but the voice of reason eventually won, so I resumed walking. Over the years, I have learned a lot about myself, cows, and anxiety.

As silly as it seems, cows provide great lessons about anxiety. If I surprised a cow, she would run away a few steps, and there would be a ripple effect, with other cows doing the same. When the cows no longer sensed a threat, they would resume quietly grazing. The easy movement of anxiety through groups comes from survival instincts, helping animals and people escape danger.[1]

Whether bovine or human, anxiety is the response to a real or perceived threat.[2] Anxiety influences our physical, psychological, and emotional functioning so we can more readily escape danger.[3] One problem is that our body doesn't know the threat difference between a real stampede or a difficult conversation. Acute and chronic stressors activate the same physiological process.[4] Frequent triggering of this process, which is meant for emergencies, is exhausting and not sustainable.[5]

Unlike cows, which quickly return to a relaxed state, we tend to get stuck thinking about potential threats.[6] This continues the stress response. Chronic anxiety has set up residence in our world and is impossible to avoid as it spreads like a contagion from person to person.[7] Ongoing stress depletes resilience and sustainability. Anxiety always will have a place in life, so we need to learn how to return to calm after the stress response is triggered.

The good news is that we can promote inner peace to influence anxiety's pull.[8] Let's look at perspectives, skills, and activities to decrease anxiety. We will consider strategies to defuse emotional triggers and create inner peace. As we do this for ourselves, we also decrease anxiety in our families and teams. Small changes in how we think create space to breathe and enjoy life's goodness. We can produce our own calm and be an oasis in the anxiety storm.

//

Resilience at Work: Imagine . . .

What a day! Nonstop demands and emotionally charged moments! The second you arrive home, exhaustion starts to hit. With a sigh, you replay difficult moments, while tomorrow looms in the back of your mind. But stop! You remember this is the time to relax, rejuvenate, and reconnect with close people. So, you take a moment to be still, give yourself a mental hug, and let go of stress. A smile lifts your soul, and peace fills the quiet space. You embrace the moment to enjoy the pieces of life beyond your helping role.

//

Strengthen Self to Decrease Pressures

We can increase calm by strengthening our sense of self while remaining connected with others. Self-differentiation is key to regulating anxiety. On the contrary, focus on relationship pressures leads us away from being the calm individuals we strive to be. Emphasis on acceptance reduces emotional separation and lessens the steady barrage of stress. Rick and Dave, nurses in busy team settings, demonstrate the impact of self-differentiation on anxiety.

Rick, an emergency nurse, is passionate about helping people. He feels happiest when everyone else is happy, so he spends a lot of energy trying to make others happy. Bouncing between helping patients and encouraging unhappy coworkers, he makes every shift an emotional marathon. Rick's inability to draw a line between his own emotions and those of others chronically increases his anxiety to high levels.

Dave, an ICU nurse, also is driven to help others and cares deeply about people. While encountering others' emotions, he remembers to be grounded in purpose and principles. Yes, the world is more pleasant when everyone is happy, but he knows he can't control others' feelings. This emotional boundary enables Dave to be a calm presence. Awareness of the boundary between his and other people's emotions decreases his anxiety and increases sustainability.

> *The most important distinction anyone can ever make in their life is between who they are as an individual and their connection with others.* —Anné Linden

Dave and Rick both bring important skills to their roles, but their different perceptions of self dramatically affect sustainability. Rick's emphasis on togetherness over a sense of self increases anxiety. Ironically, his lower self-differentiation makes it harder to have healthy connections, because stress gets in the way.[9] The focus on other people's emotions creates pressures that push him in a variety of directions.

Dave's journey is less confused by other people's emotions. He is able to be present with other people's emotions while remaining purpose focused. His ability to differentiate from others gives him the emotional space to process and recover from challenges. Dave makes decisions based on what is important, rather than on concerns of how others will respond. A stronger sense of self helps Dave connect with others while journeying on his individual path.

The constant tug-of-war between individuality and togetherness is a primary source of the anxiety we experience.[10] Our natural drive to be unique individuals competes with the perceived need to be like others in order to be accepted. Relationship uncertainty amplifies stress. We are more likely to absorb and adapt to other people's anxieties while being ruled by emotions.[11] Concern about acceptance leads us to live more from pressures and vulnerabilities than from values and purpose.[12]

MAKE THE FORCE BE WITH YOU

We can use force for good even if we aren't a part of the Star Wars saga. The pressures we experience come from a web of internal and external sources. While many are beyond our control, we do influence how those pressures shape our thoughts, decisions, and responses. Consider the pressures of your role and mindfully discern:

- What is unfair or unrealistic?

- What pressures do you create, and how do they relate to a need for acceptance?

- What pressures can you see differently so they become a motivator rather than a drain?

We can change the cyclone of anxiety by putting a stop to unrealistic expectations and seeing pressure for what it is—a force trying to move us in a certain way. Let's influence those forces so they help rather than hinder our journey.

Emphasis on how we connect rather than on who we are also can lead to overfunctioning. It takes on the disguise of helping others but creates dependence, increases anxiety, and reduces sustainability.[13] Rick's efforts to keep everyone happy move him to cross healthy boundaries. He tries to take on other people's responsibilities, including their emotional well-being. Rick's overfunctioning diminishes sustainability and the abilities of others to handle their own challenges.

Helping others does not mean we give up our individuality. Nor are we to diminish other people's sense of self. We promote self-differentiation for ourselves and others by remaining grounded in what is important and being guided by our core self. Our core self is the thoughtful, mature part of who we are that prods us to do better and stand for what we believe.[14]

Living from our core self and purpose decreases the influence of pressures. A stronger sense of self increases authenticity and inner peace. This is far more stable than relying on ever-changing circumstances and responses of others. One of the best gifts we can offer is to strengthen our sense of self to provide a calm presence. By identifying what triggers emotional responses, we take a leap closer to this reality.

Voices from the Field: Start with personal growth and care.

"Before I can really help others, I need to start with my own self-care. How I am doing affects how well I can connect with other people. Personal growth, mindfulness, social gatherings, exercise, and sleep all influence how well I can control my own emotions—one of the most important and difficult tasks of helping others." Isabel, Mental Health Provider, Honduras

Recognize and Defuse Emotional Triggers

We can decrease anxiety by making emotional triggers less reactive. If we fail to deal with our own triggers, we experience more anxiety and increase stress for others. Consider the following scenario with Derek and Maren, coworkers in a busy clinic.

While crossing the hall, Derek called out to Maren, but she didn't respond. Derek felt ignored and became irritated. He was still annoyed when talking with Maren later, but he didn't say anything. She felt the tension and became anxious when he was around. Even if Derek lets it go for a while, the next time Maren does something similar, the trigger likely will be quicker and more intense. Derek is headed on an escalating anxiety ride and dragging others along.

Self-awareness can help Derek function less anxiously. Emotional triggers often are related to the need for connection, accompanied by lower self-differentiation.[15] We all have emotional triggers, but they vary in reactivity. Let's rewind to the interaction and consider an alternative response that's based on an awareness of the emotional trigger and a stronger sense of self.

Derek knows being ignored sets off an emotional reaction that shuts down his ability to reason. After Maren didn't respond, he noticed that his heart rate sped up and his mind started to yell. He took a breath, remembered there were better ways to respond, and decreased his emotional reaction.

Derek recentered his sense of self on important values and purpose rather than Maren's response. This paused his reactivity so he could recognize there may have been many reasons why Maren didn't reply. Increased self-regulation made room for reason and creativity. He either dropped the need to discuss it or asked Maren about her lack of response in a calm manner. Derek defused the emotional trigger and engaged in a healthier process, thus reducing anxiety.

We always have the choice to decrease or add to a group's anxiety and negativity. If we fail to regulate our own emotions, we become like a superconductor passing anxiety through the group.[16] As we regulate our emotions to decrease our anxiety, we also decrease group anxiety.[17] We can move toward a calm journey when we notice emotional triggers and choose healthy perspectives.

STRATEGIES TO DEFUSE EMOTIONAL TRIGGERS

1. Write down behaviors, comments, or interactions that affect you emotionally. Often, triggers are related to how we see ourselves or are connected to actions we feel violate important virtues and values.

2. Think about why such actions are triggers and come up with a simple reminder to interrupt the emotional response.

3. Take it a step further by identifying unhelpful behavior patterns that follow emotional triggers.

4. Pick a calming word or positive statement that helps you focus on what is important and promotes self-differentiation.

5. Describe responses that better represent you at your best, balanced self.

6. Imagine yourself responding in ways you see as ideal during difficult situations. Neuroplasticity, our brains' ability to change, allows us to develop new ways of thinking and

behaving at any age.[18] When we imagine different behaviors, we actually increase our ability to respond in those ways during emotionally heated moments.

Choose Your Life Perspective

A Chinese folktale about a man whose axe went missing illustrates the power of perspective. The man looked behind his shed and under the wheelbarrow but couldn't find his axe. As his frustration grew, he happened to see his neighbor's son. He suspected the boy took it, because he thought the boy looked like a thief, walked like a thief, and talked like a thief. Later that day the man found his axe in the valley where he had left it. When he saw his neighbor's son again, the boy looked, walked, and talked like any other boy.[19] How we see the world affects how we experience the world.

Voices from the Field: See the positive.

"The need is overwhelming. I try to see how small actions have an impact on such big problems. Helping one life at a time is important, because there are multipliers out there—people who do a lot and make big differences." Judith, International Services Coordinator, Honduras

Positive perspectives counter negative influences that seem to pervade life. Positive emotions move our brain into a more proactive, open, and optimistic way of functioning.[20] As powerful as they are, mindsets geared toward gratitude, hope, and joy don't just happen. Intentional efforts develop such attitudes.

I want to be clear about something: I am not suggesting we put on a happy face and pretend to feel a certain way. I am referring to the possibility of choosing to experience joy, gratitude, hope, and peace. Sometimes we need medical help to change how we feel, but our perspective does influence how we experience life.[21]

"Pain is inevitable, but misery is optional," wrote Tim Hansel after breaking his back in a climbing fall. He explained, "We cannot avoid pain, but we can avoid joy . . . Joy is simple (not to be confused with easy). At any moment in life, we have at least two options, and one of them is to choose an attitude of gratitude, a posture of grace, a commitment to joy."[22]

Joy, gratitude, and hope are part of a mindset, a way of being that can march into the midst of suffering with a stubborn refusal to let darkness dominate. We can grow a joyful, grateful, and hopeful perspective, or we can get caught in the trap of waiting for it to happen. Vera and Vi, women I visited while I was their pastor, provided great examples of contrasting perspectives. The ninety-five-year-old women resided in the same care center, but lived worlds apart.

Vera always greeted me with a big smile and complimented me, saying, "You have such nice teeth." She went on to say, "The staff here are so wonderful! I am so thankful for them." Visits ended with hugs and a "Thank you!"

A short walk down the colorless hall led to a very different scene. As soon as Vi saw me, she started her complaints. "Staff ignore me. The food is terrible. My family doesn't do enough." Visits ended with a final complaint: "Don't take so long to come see me again."

Life was hard for both women, but Vera's perspective helped her connect with others and enjoy life. Emphasis on positives loosened the grip of suffering. People like Vera can inspire us to choose a more positive perspective, and people like Vi show us why doing so is important.

We can give ourselves permission to experience joy, gratitude, peace, and hope, especially when the world seems heavy. There is no world of suffering that does not also contain the goodness of life. Archbishop Desmond Tutu said, "We are fragile creatures, and it is from this weakness, not despite it, that we discover the possibility of true joy."[23] Suffering and positives such as joy are not paradoxical, but coexist in our imperfect world.

Life's grand mix of experiences provides the landscape for our journeys. How we perceive those experiences determines who we are. In difficult roles, especially when suffering is involved, we can choose how to respond. Be intentional about reflecting what is important. We can respond to difficult experiences in ways that invite gratitude, hope, and joy to be part of the journey. Fostering inner peace provides windows to see such beauty beyond the difficult.

Increase Outer Calm with Inner Peace

Inner peace can seem like a distant dream as we consider the chaos swirling around us. Do any of the following scenarios describe your work helping others?

- Trying to herd a group of cats with a dog watching.

- Leading an expedition with only a roll of dental floss.

- Holding a relay race with turtles while unable to see the finish line.

- Gathering a herd of sheep because there might be a storm, even though there isn't a cloud in the sky.

- Trying to teach the dog and herd of cats to rock climb with dental floss while racing turtles during a storm as the sheep run wild.

Our world includes an ever-present whirlwind of anxiety. A global pandemic, social unrest, frequent natural disasters, political polarization. Anxiety is flying all over the place. Every moment of any given day there's an abundance of stress ready to fatigue and sideline good people working hard to help others.

Voices from the Field: See the effects of stress.

"Ever since I was a child, I was a caregiver. I wanted to help my parents and sister, but there were times it was overwhelming. The stress affected my whole life. I was tired, sad, lonely, anxious, angry, and unhealthy. I knew I had to do something for my own survival." Jill, Family Caregiver, United States

Imagine if life could be characterized more by peace than chaos? A serene mountain lake on a sunny day, rather than an ocean during a hurricane. There is much we cannot control in the world, but we can influence the role of anxiety in our own lives. Fostering internal peace provides a lens with which we see more of the world's goodness and possibilities.[24]

Activities promoting calm help us move out of the fight-or-flight mode anxiety provokes. We were created to function predominantly in a more relaxed mode, so it is in this state that we can think rationally, learn more, approach problems creatively, and work more sustainably.[25] Efforts promoting calm change our relationship with emotions. Inner peace helps us approach feelings with curiosity rather than negative judgments that increase their impact.[26]

The world's chaos may make it hard to believe peace is possible, but we each carry the capacity to promote inner peace.[27] Ancient wisdom and contemporary research affirm this as not only possible but also valuable to overall health.[28] The inner calm we create positively shapes our own lives and the world around us.[29]

Want to experience a life that resembles that serene mountain lake more than a stormy ocean? Give yourself permission to differentiate from the world's anxieties. Embrace a different way of being. Focus on the core of who you are and be a calming presence even when the world seems chaotic.

Add simple activities to increase calm to your daily routine. Intentionally make peace a habit and stress an occasional byproduct of life. Encourage pain's energy to move on from your life, rather than holding on to it.[30] You can add the following activities to your stress-reduction kit:

Give yourself timeouts: Set aside a few minutes each day to allow yourself to be still—to let go of anxiety and the compulsion to do more. Mindfully connect with yourself. Spiritually connect with God. The more we do this quiet work, the more we can regulate our responses when anxiety is rising.[31]

- Practice mindfulness: Draw in a deep breath and exhale slowly, letting go of anxiety. Breathe in calm. Breathe out stress. With closed eyes, pay attention to your breathing and heart beating. Allow yourself to simply be. Take note of emotions and feelings. Don't amplify or undermine; simply acknowledge them. This is not the moment to fix anything—it is a moment to check-in.[32]

- Pray.

- Meditate (guided or silent).

- Practice yoga.

> *We all have, lying deep within us, in our hearts and in our very bones, a capacity for a dynamic, vital, sustaining inner peacefulness and well-being.*[33] —Jon Kabat-Zinn

Breathe with a calming word: Think of a word or two that brings calm. Now pair it with a deep breath. For example, my word is "Jesu." To promote calm, I close my eyes, take a deep breath, and silently say, "Jesu." Inhale for four seconds and exhale for six seconds while silently saying your word. Deep breathing is an easy win-win, as it promotes relaxation and communication between different parts of the brain.[34] Try this before every appointment and meeting, or whenever you want to create inner calm.

Hug yourself like a butterfly: No joke—give yourself a hug. Like certain breathing exercises, warm, gentle touch activates nerves, helping our body relax. Offer yourself a butterfly hug, and increase the calming effect by alternately tapping each arm while embracing yourself.[35] If you are with other people and prefer to do something less conspicuous, alternately tap each leg. This bilateral stimulation calms our nervous system and promotes balanced brain functioning.

Voices from the Field: Know you aren't alone.

"I feel more confident when I pray before doing anything important. Praying gives me peace and reminds me that God is with me." Anthony, Medical Student, Honduras

---

Nourish spirituality: We are part of something much bigger than ourselves. Get in touch with and nourish your spirituality to remember this. Different from religion, spirituality is turning ourselves toward a greater power and finding unity in a purpose outside of ourselves. We can discover uplifting warmth, contentment, and joy in experiencing what we cannot reduce to explanation.[36] Spirituality helps us search for answers to life's mysteries and moves us toward meaning after difficult experiences.[37]

As we remember that there is so much beyond our understanding, we also are reminded of our limitations. We are more able to let go of what we can't change and allow ourselves to not be a god, but let the divine work. Pray, study sacred writings, listen to inspirational music, and gather with others to worship. When we nourish our spirituality, we connect with natural and divine forces, continually creating hopeful possibilities.

Voices from the Field: Connect with your spirituality.

"My relationship with God has been a moral compass and source of strength. When I nurture that relationship, I have found that I am much stronger than I ever thought. I feel like I'm doing God's work. Even when it is tough and I've had a bad day, I remember, "You're doing what you're supposed to do, and you are strong enough." Raye, Veterinarian, United States

Provoke playfulness: Don't forget to play! Exercise, sleep, nutritious eating, and other self-care tasks decrease the toll of stress.[38] When you hike in nature, it's easy to enjoy the benefits of exercise and mindfulness. Immerse yourself in a creative hobby, vacation, or family games to experience simple joys. Encourage laughter. Delight in the beauty and blessings that can be easy to overlook. Combine basic self-care with playfulness to create a resilience dynamic duo.

In a world filled with stress, we can choose to walk in an anxious frenzy or experience something different. We need to consciously get out of the world's anxiety tornado. Time and effort put toward self-discovery and healthy living make everything more sustainable. When it comes to anxiety, the choices we make will either increase or decrease the stress in our own life and the lives of others we interact with.

Decrease Group Anxiety

We can be a source of calm by standing firm in our individuality amid pressures.[39] However, remaining non-anxious can be difficult, because anxiety is transmitted so easily within groups. Emotional triangles are among the biggest culprits when it comes to spreading anxiety. The pull to participate in anxious sharing with others is strong and countered only by self-differentiation. Consider the influence of self-differentiation and emotional triangles on group anxiety with examples from nurses Rick and Dave.

Rick is very perceptive to how everyone is feeling and wants to fix things when anyone is unhappy. Ginny talked with Rick about a frustrating moment she had with Janet. Rick became anxious because Ginny was upset, and he talked with John, another colleague. His effort to decrease anxiety did the opposite. Despite good intentions, Rick created emotional triangles that elevated team anxiety and dysfunction. Forming emotional triangles reveals a lack of self-differentiation and decreases sustainability.[40]

If just one person can remain connected to group members without sharing anxiety, it will decrease group anxiety.[41] Dave also cares about his team but remembers his emotions can be different. He focuses on purpose rather than feelings. When Ashley talked with him about her frustrations with Tom, Dave calmly listened and encouraged her to talk to Tom. He provided support while staying attentive to his own perspective and emotions. Dave didn't share the frustrations with others, so he decreased group anxiety.

STRATEGIES TO LOWER GROUP ANXIETY

1. Increase emotional differentiation and practice mindfulness. Return focus toward purpose when group anxiety tugs at your attention.

2. Expand awareness of and disrupt social processes that move anxiety through groups—for example, emotional triangles.

3. Get perspective on team problems from resources outside of the group first. If you need to address a problem within the team, do so as non-anxiously as possible.

4. Stay connected and choose to be a calm presence. How we position ourselves determines whether we are a negative or positive influence.

We always have a choice whether to increase or decrease group anxiety. We can be live wires, easily sharing anxiety, or insulators grounded in thoughtful purpose. Our positive influence grows as we increase the ability to regulate emotions and decrease anxiety. The peace we foster within brings goodness to others as well.

Journey with Peace

What does peace mean to you? It is easy to think of peace as the absence of anxiety, conflict, violence, and war. Peace really is so much more, and it applies to individual as well as collective life. We may feel peace while walking in the woods or sitting around a campfire with others. We can experience peace in myriad ways, but only when we find personal peace can we share peace with others.

Individual and collective peace is the overwhelming presence of goodness despite brokenness and struggles. The Hebrew concept *shalom*, often translated as "peace," means total well-being, tranquility, and security.[42] It comes from divine blessing and is a manifestation of God's grace. Shalom does not come in the absence of troubles, but promotes wellbeing even when conflict and difficulties exist.

My hope for you is shalom. Amid the challenges of caring for people, may you let go of the anxieties swirling around you and embrace the deep abiding peace you carry within. Be distinctly you while being connected and caring for others. Peace is a gift we can carry within and share even in times of challenge.

Now that we have looked at ways to decrease anxiety, we will consider strategies for handling conflict to promote sustainability. Disagreements certainly can shake up our sense of calm, but they don't need to rattle our resilience. Get ready to expand your conflict resolution skillset so disagreements don't take as much of an emotional toll. Conflict often creates storms on its own, but we can face differences with hope and peace.

GUIDE TO THRIVE STRATEGIES

1. Increase self-differentiation:

   a. Remember you can be in connection with others while remaining an individual with a unique set of goals, values, experiences, emotions, and ideas.

   b. Increase the ability to remain non-anxious and regulate personal emotions.

2. Discern and decrease emotional triggers.

3. Describe and mentally rehearse responses you want to have to difficult situations.

4. Give yourself permission to experience joy, gratitude, peace, and hope, and intentionally foster perspectives that promote these healthy virtues.

5. Practice mindfulness and make time for quiet moments daily.

6. Integrate a breathing exercise throughout your day and pair it with a calming word.

7. Give yourself a butterfly hug.

8. Nourish spirituality and embrace being part of something bigger than yourself.

9. Promote playfulness and self-care.

10. Increase understanding of social processes and develop skills to stop participation in group anxiety.

---- **Discussion Questions** ----

What pressures do you see creating anxiety?

Can you share a time when you were able to decrease anxiety in a situation?

What will you do to increase inner peace?

How does anxiety affect groups?

What can you do to help decrease anxiety in your family, team, or organization?

Would you like to discuss any other ideas from the chapter?

Chapter 6

DEAL WITH CONFLICT

We decrease anxiety and create new possibilities
when we take the sting out of conflict.

Perceive Conflict's Possibilities

Conflict can rattle our journey even when we have the most virtuous intentions. Our veterinary staff experienced this when Carla brought her dog in for a routine exam. All was going well until Carla went to check out in the lobby. Surrounded by other clients with their animals waiting for appointments, she yelled at staff, "Why are you treating me this way!" Then she wept. Carla's unexpected outburst left veterinary staff shocked and wondering what they had done wrong.

Days later when I saw Carla, she apologized for her behavior. With tears in her eyes, she explained that just before the appointment, she had learned her husband was having an affair with her best friend. We can relate to her emotional vulnerability after such a discovery, but staff were not aware of her personal problems and bore the brunt of her fury.

Unexpected conflict can shake us to the core. For many of us, just seeing the word "conflict" creates anxiety. Often times, we don't have the extra energy to deal with disagreements, so they take more of a toll

113

than expected. Daily disagreements rarely reach catastrophic levels, yet they can turn us inside out and wear us down.

We may wish for a life without conflict, but reality reminds us that disagreements are inevitable. If you think about it, conflict litters everyone's family tree, affecting the vitality of present-day branches. Injustice, war, oppression, and other conflictual forces determined the soil quality in which family trees grew. How has conflict shaped your story?

Due to conflict's enduring presence, how we perceive and deal with it influences sustainability. If we can see conflict with a positive spin, we decrease anxiety and improve our ability to handle difficult situations. We can disrupt unhelpful conflict habits and use practical strategies to decrease its toll even more. We'll also look at difficult dynamics and consider how to help others without taking on their conflict. Successfully navigating conflict's storms begins with getting a grip on how we see its role in our journey.

Resilience at Work: Imagine . . .

"Today is going to be a good day!" You smile and greet people as the day begins. Someone stops you, asking for advice on how to handle a disagreement. You listen, provide support, and refrain from taking on her battle. Time slips by, and the day feels smooth until angry criticism puts a stop to your rhythm. It is unexpected and hurtful. You take a deep breath, give yourself a mental hug, and determine whether the problem should be dealt with at that moment. Although conflict took you by surprise, you know you have the strength and skills to face it.

Grow Your Capacity for Calm and Resolution

Our perception of conflict determines the toll it will take and the possibilities for resolution. The mixture of anxiety and conflict is more likely to close doors than to inspire creative responses. Imagine walking down a brightly lit hallway. You see a number of doors open and pictures artistically spaced on the walls. Images of people smiling, flowers blooming, and animals romping catch your eye. Suddenly, an angry creature stands in your way. The bright images disappear, and doors close. The angry creature dominates what you see, think, and feel.

When we just see conflict as a threat, it becomes like an angry creature taking over the journey. Anxiety sets off our fight-or-flight system, hampering the ability to respond rationally and creatively.[1] Fear slams shut the doors to possibilities. We can reduce stress and expand potential for healthy change by seeing conflict differently. We continue to see the brightly lit walls, colorful pictures, and open doors even when disagreements appear threatening.

Consider the following perceptions to decrease conflict's emotional toll:

Conflict is a natural part of life: History is littered with clashes affecting people on every continent and arising from our fundamental needs for connection and individuality.[2] As long as we are working with people who have their own perceptions, desires, and stories, we will have to deal with conflict.[3]

Conflict resolution promotes wellness: We may feel the pull to avoid disagreements, but unresolved conflict leads to destructive patterns within families, teams, and organizations.[4]

Dissension that has been carried over time eventually erupts with more volatility than if it had been addressed from the beginning.[5] Choose your battles well, but also consider how old battles inform today's journey.

Conflict helps us discover greater truths: We always enter conflict with only a portion of the truth.[6] Similar to coming upon an iceberg, we may think we see it all, but there is much below the surface we don't see. Disagreements can help us learn more about ourselves, others, and the world.

Conflict can be transformative: Ideally, conflict promotes healthy change and opportunities. Just think about the social justice and other advancements resulting from conflict. We expand our ability to deal with disagreements when we see conflict as a force that potentially leads to new, healthier possibilities.[7]

Voices from the Field: Believe conflict can create new possibilities.

"Sometimes, we need to disrupt the donkey cart. When I started, the team was dysfunctional, so I took on organizational realignment. I assigned more women who showed skills to leadership positions. This caused quite a stir. After reorganizing and supporting new leaders, we had a much stronger team." Judith, International Services Coordinator, Honduras

---

If you think about it, conflict isn't the problem. How people deal with conflict makes it problematic. When we see conflict only as an obstacle, we decrease our ability to problem-solve.[8] However, when we see conflict as a natural part of life and a way to promote positive change based on deeper truths, we are better able to respond in proactive ways.

We rarely choose the conflicts that disrupt life, but we do determine how to respond. Holocaust survivor Viktor Frankl noted, "Everything can be taken from a (person) but one thing: the last of the human freedoms—to choose one's attitude in any given set of circumstances, to choose one's own way."[9]

How we respond influences whether disagreements will be constructive or destructive. We will enhance either connection or separation, pursue justice or oppression, and foster new discovery or rigid thinking.[10] Conflict always involves more than one person, but we can control only our responses. While it is often easier to point out other people's shortcomings, we all have unhealthy conflict habits that create barriers and close doors.

Perception is the first step in opening the doors of resolution and reconciliation when conflict steps in the way. Let's say we now see conflict as a natural part of life that can promote greater truth and transformative change. We then can take the next step toward dealing with conflict constructively by identifying and replacing unhelpful behavior patterns.

> *Peace is not merely a distant goal that we seek, but a means by which we arrive at that goal.* —Martin Luther King, Jr.

Recognize and Replace Unhelpful Conflict Habits

We may be tempted to point at other people when conflict arises, but we'll be more effective if we work on disrupting our own conflict habits. Consider an example with Mary and Jenna, employees at the Community Health Center. Parents holding infants, small children sitting on laps, and adults of all ages filled the waiting room. Staff rushed between appointments, grabbing bites from lunches on occasion.

Amid the busyness, Mary looked for some medicine she had just seen Jenna using. Frazzled and tired, she blamed Jenna for the missing vial. After angrily reprimanding Jenna, she found it hidden behind her own microscope but didn't say anything. Jenna, feeling hurt and angry, shared her frustrations with Carl, who then avoided Mary. Each person in this emotional triangle fell into conflict habits and increased anxiety.

Mary, Jenna, and Carl have unique individual journeys, but their conflict behaviors are common habits.[11] We all have automatic responses to fall back on when stressed, even when we know they are not the most effective. Identifying unhelpful behaviors provides the opportunity to develop healthier responses.

We benefit most by concentrating on our own functioning, but awareness of behavior patterns can help us understand others as well. Focusing on behaviors rather than individuals helps us address tough situations and deal more effectively with difficult social dynamics. Recognizing the imperfect humanity behind unhealthy behavior patterns slows down the emotional leap to defensiveness.

Like any habit, conflict habits are tough to change, especially when we are tired and stressed. Old habits may never disappear completely, but the more we rehearse and use healthier responses, the easier it gets.

Look at the following conflict habits to discern which you tend to use and how to change them.

Blame: Projecting blame reduces the capacity to consider other per-spectives and work toward solutions.[12] It is an easy go-to behavior that does not require self-examination. Or, if we tend to blame ourselves, then we don't hold others accountable. Either way, blame increases anxiety and divisiveness. As illustrated by Mary blaming Jenna, such behavior obstructs dealing with the actual problem and damages relationships.[13]

Change the Habit: Catch yourself when blame jumps to mind. Think about mutual responsibility and the challenges that need to be overcome. Rather than attributing blame, focus on what needs to be changed and create possible solutions. Mary could have avoided conflict if, before accusing Jenna, she had looked or asked staff to help her find the medicine.

Emotional triangles: When there is anxiety between two people, one or both may focus on a third person or group.[14] The intent is to decrease anxiety, but it actually increases anxiety, dysfunction, and negativity.[15] Jenna drawing Carl into her frustration may have momentarily decreased her stress, but it increased tension between Carl and Mary. If Carl shares concerns about the two with other staff, he creates more triangles and increases group reactivity.[16]

Change the Habit: Stop talking about others. When frustrated with someone, talk directly with that person or get perspective from someone outside of the group. Jenna could have increased group functioning if she had talked calmly with Mary or talked with a wise friend not connected to the clinic.

Avoidance: We all need to consider what battles are worth taking on, but to chronically avoid difficult people or issues doesn't produce resolution. Carl's avoidance of Mary will only make it harder for both of them and will negatively influence staff dynamics. While it may be temporarily helpful to distance from conflict, to do so repeatedly increases anxiety and reduces the ability to handle difficult situations.[17]

Change the Habit: Ground your sense of self on important values and purpose to find courage to deal with difficult situations. Decrease anxiety and expand communication skills to face challenges in ways you can feel good about. Give yourself some time to discern whether you need to follow up, and then strategize how to do so. If Carl recognized that he didn't need to take on Jenna's emotions or try to fix the problem, he would not have been compelled to avoid Mary.

Win-lose approach: This method denies the multitude of possibilities for collaboration and transformation. It sets a more aggressive, divisive tone, because the goal becomes conquering rather than learning and growing.[18] The perspective focuses on winners and losers. Nobody wants to be a loser. Mary and Jenna's failure to talk demonstrates this approach and the inability to see how conflict provides opportunities for growth.

Change the Habit: Before diving into a competitive mode, remember there may be possibilities you can't easily see. For Mary or Jenna, initiating a respectful conversation could have increased the likelihood of a positive outcome. Think in terms of both/and rather than either/or to promote solutions benefiting everyone.[19] Foster creativity to expand win-win thought processes.

Quick overreactivity: High emotionality makes it difficult to respond rationally, because the focus is on anxiety rather than the problem.[20] As long as Mary, Jenna, and Carl focus on emotions, it will be difficult to reduce stress. Higher levels of anxiety diminish our ability to keep perspective and creatively work toward solutions. (Due to the many challenges it causes, high emotional reactivity is covered in this chapter's *Navigate the Difficult* section.)

Change the Habit: Increase self-differentiation and the ability to regulate emotions. If Mary, Jenna, and Carl had recognized their own emotional responsibility and taken time to think about the problem, they could have decreased the anxiety for the whole staff.

Once we identify unhelpful behaviors, we can change negative patterns. Define how you hope to handle differences, and imagine yourself responding to conflict in ways that reflect your best, balanced self. Give yourself some "You can do it!" encouragement to use healthy principles and discover the potential positives of conflict.

BRING YOUR BEST TO CONFLICT

As you consider how to deal with conflict, include the work you have done articulating important principles, values, and purpose. Recall your description of yourself at your healthy best and integrate that into dealing with differences. Remember your emotional triggers and the ways you can defuse them.

- Describe how you want to respond in moments of conflict. What does this look like physically, emotionally, and cognitively? Be specific.

- What virtues do you hope to convey?

Mentally rehearse responses. Practice calmly handling disagreements in front of a mirror or with a trusted person to discover unhelpful body language or tone of voice. As you do so, affirm the strength you have to handle difficult situations. Repetition will make it easier to respond calmly even when surprised by conflict.

Use Care-Full Strategies

Conflict-resolution strategies promote care-full responses. Pressures for immediate resolution are common in today's world and can derail thoughtful replies. First responders Brenda and Luke know the benefit of quick responses while helping others, but found the same doesn't apply to conflict. The team had just returned from a multivehicle accident. Cold temperatures and snow had added to the challenge of rescuing people who had injuries ranging from minor to critical. Exhausted team members dropped into chairs, mentally willing the shift to end.

Brenda, the squad supervisor, checked emails and discovered one marked urgent. The message detailed a new schedule policy requiring more on-call time and requested her to inform employees as soon as possible. She knew there would be grumbling and dreaded telling her crew, but she decided to get it over with. Brenda called the group together and read the email about schedule changes.

Luke, like everyone else, was exhausted and upset. He confronted Brenda in front of the team, yelling, "You are such a crappy leader! You never have our backs!" Brenda was shocked and wanted to yell at

Luke, but instead she marched into her office, slamming the door. As brief as the encounter was, it rattled the team for a long time.

As you look at the following strategies, consider what would have helped Brenda and Luke. What strategies could be especially helpful for you? Keep in mind—culture and context do matter. They establish norms that determine how to understand and deal with conflict. We need to move outside of unhealthy cultural norms, but we also need to determine how to do so effectively, with respect.

Manage time proactively: A move away from seeking instant resolution can be difficult in a society used to quick fixes. However, time used well moves us from reactivity to thoughtful proactivity. Create space to process conflict by communicating an intent to address the problem at a specified time. Others may not perceive the value of doing this, but let them know the matter is important enough to allow time. The ability to approach a problem with rational thinking and creativity will be a gift to everyone involved.

USE TIME AS AN ALLY, NOT AN ESCAPE

When dealing with conflict, choose a day and time most likely to produce positive results. Proactively use time to do the following:

- Decrease anxiety.
- Ground yourself in personal and organizational values, virtues, and purpose.
- Define the problem.

- Gather information.
- Develop potential solutions and responses.
- Practice responses that reflect your best, balanced self.

Start with common ground: Finding common ground helps make everyone comfortable and promotes cooperation.[21] This can be a shared purpose or connection defined by relationship, organization, or society that promotes a focus on shared interests and reduces a win-lose perspective. Cooperation based on mutually beneficial goals is far more constructive than pushing a position that's helpful only for a few.[22] Return often to shared purpose and goals.

Listen actively: Active listening involves pausing your own thoughts to listen and then repeating what you heard.[23] As simple as this seems, it is difficult because we seldom listen without analyzing, comparing, or developing responses. Repeating what you heard does not imply you agree, but it conveys that you care enough to listen. Explain time limitations at the beginning of the conversation to promote focused listening.

Clarify calmly: Clarify issues with open-ended questions rather than assuming everyone is dealing with the same issue. Concisely define what you see as the point of conflict. Specific explanations decrease defensiveness and enable problem solving.[24] Communicate as non-anxiously as possible to help the other person(s) understand your perspective. Do not assume they see problems the same way you do. Since there's conflict, it's likely they perceive the situation differently and have little or no awareness of your perspective.

Use "I" statements: Speak only for yourself. When we take responsibility for our own feelings, thoughts, and experiences, we are less likely to blame others and come across as aggressive.[25] For example, saying "I feel sad" rather than "You make me sad" is far more likely to lead to positive problem solving. "I" statements focus more on your response to what has happened, rather than on another person's actions, and they are more likely to be heard because they don't attack others' sense of self.

Focus on the positive: Foster a constructive perspective by focusing on the positive when possible. Identify what you see as good rather than being stuck on what is wrong. Positivity promotes open conversation and cooperation.[26] A rant on the negatives can become oppressive and diminish hopes for reaching a resolution.[27] Giving positive direction and reinforcement is much more effective.

Pay attention to nonverbal cues: *How* we talk may communicate more than what we say. Be aware of body language and tone of voice. When feeling defensive or aggressive, what postures or verbal habits do you tend to fall into? Ask a safe person to describe how you usually respond, or videotape role-playing situations. Replace aggressive or defensive nonverbal cues with ones that communicate calm. We are more likely to convey peace when body language and voice reinforce our words.[28]

Agree when possible: Give glimpses of a win-win resolution by agreeing when you're able to do so. Common ground or purpose provides an important basis for resolution. Each time genuine agreement is expressed, it affirms all perspectives and brings movement toward cooperation.[29]

Have potential solutions, but be open to other possibilities: We can start a resolution process with potential actions in mind, but it's just a starting point. If we get too committed to our initial ideas, we are less likely to listen and engage in mutual problem solving. A tolerance of ambiguity promotes openness to unexpected solutions and creative thinking.

Use Mediation: In an ideal world, we can resolve conflict and even turn it into opportunities for growth. Unfortunately, life doesn't always work out this way. Mediation encourages understanding and openness in high-conflict situations.[30] If the conflict feels unsafe or threatening, please get appropriate help immediately.

What strategies do you think Brenda and Luke could have used to promote resolution rather than conflict? As a leader, Brenda had the responsibility to direct the process with integrity, representing the organization positively. Luke also had a duty to interact with maturity and respect. Both would have benefited from taking time to think and grounding their responses in important principles. Responses driven by a common goal, such as team and client wellness, are more likely than emotional reactions to produce transformative resolution.

We can deal with disagreements in healthy ways when we are grounded in what is important and have handy conflict strategies. We positively influence teams when we regulate our emotional responses and believe conflict can lead to healthy change. Different dynamics can make conflict trickier to handle, but there are ways to navigate the more difficult twists on our journey.

Navigate the Difficult

Have you ever faced any of the following conflict complications?

- Someone's response seemed out of proportion with what happened.

- You felt you had to be careful around someone, because their reactions to even simple challenges were unnerving.

- Conflict was dealt with and resolved, but the other person seems to be stuck in the disagreement.

- You were afraid to deal with an issue, because the person you need to confront has authority and may make life harder for you.

Such scenarios make conflict seem like facing a mountain rather than a bump in the path. The most common difficult dynamics people have shared with me include dealing with highly emotional people and power differences. A glimpse at each scenario can clarify what strategies are most helpful and make the mountain seem smaller.

Voices from the Field: Resist taking on other people's conflicts.

"I deal with conflict every day, whether it is getting someone to follow safety regulations or someone is yelling at people because they took too much food. People in the vulnerable population I work with can get aggressive, and you don't know when it's going to happen. I try to get people to take responsibility for their own conflict and behaviors, but it isn't easy." Scott, Nonprofit Leader, United States

Handle High Emotional Reactivity with Calm

Does it ever feel like someone you deal with is about to explode, but you don't know what will set their fuse? Even the calmest people face times when it is hard to remain non-anxious, but people living with heightened emotions experience conflict more intensely.[31] They have a quick emotional reaction that overrides rational thinking.[32] The intensity of their reaction tends to be out of proportion to what has happened.

People with high emotional reactivity have difficulty returning to their emotional baseline or a state of calm. Such vulnerabilities often provoke a mix of guilt and shame, leading to a cycle of emotional reactivity. Try these useful strategies for highly reactive situations.

Regulate your own emotions: Remember that our presence influences whether anxiety decreases or increases. Mindfully validate your own emotional experience while intentionally separating your emotions from other people's emotions.[33]

Honor healthy boundaries: Highly reactive people have difficulty with boundaries, because emotional needs overcome everything else.[34] Boundaries promote sustainability for everyone, so don't change them to accommodate overreactivity. Articulate limits as non-anxiously as possible, explaining that limits promote healthy resolution.

Listen actively and validate: Don't try to talk someone out of feelings you find unreasonable, because that only exacerbates the situation.[35] Use active listening and validate the individual by finding something in their experience you can relate to. This is not the same as agreeing, but it shows care. After doing this, try to move into problem solving. Repeat active listening and validation every time emotions are on the rise.

Voices from the Field: Create positive change amid difficult dynamics.

"In nursing, there is a power differential. This can make helping others challenging and is pronounced in systems where nurses have been undermined. We create positive change when respect crosses power differences." Laurie, Nurse, United States

---

Manage Power Differences

Power differences make conflict more complicated. We may know it's important to deal with an issue, but contradicting someone else's authority can feel like jumping off a cliff and not knowing where we will land. Loyalty to an organization or cause does not mean following without a conscience.[36] Effective team members remain focused on a common purpose and thoughtfully share insights with courage, even when they differ with people who have more power. Personal and organizational values help provide guidance when we need to express a conflicting opinion.

Here are some steps provided by Ira Chaleff to intelligently counter authority:[37]

1. Understand and apply the group's mission, values, and goals to problem solving.

2. Get information to clarify the problem.

3. Determine possible solutions and repercussions.

4. Choose to comply or resist, and offer acceptable alternatives.

5. Be ready to accept personal responsibility for your choice, as there will be accountability even after following an order given by someone else.

Power differences and high emotionality increase conflict's challenges, but don't need to stop our journey. We can navigate through the challenges more easily when we remain grounded in purpose and values. As helpers, we work with a beautiful array of people who increase the possibilities for meaning and conflict. Sometimes, the people we help draw us into their conflicts. We can provide support while honoring healthy boundaries.

Help Others Deal with Conflict

We can help others deal with conflict while staying in our own yard. Reconsider the yard metaphor that illustrated limits and responsibilities. Each person has their own fenced yard containing personal responsibilities such as happiness, purpose, and well-being. Do you remember what is in your yard? Now, think about where other people's conflict belongs.

Even when we know we aren't responsible for other people's conflict, defying the pull to develop resolution is hard. We may think we are helping, but we're actually decreasing individual and group potential.[38] We increase overall group effectiveness by supporting individuals to take on their own responsibilities.

The following are tips for helping others deal with conflict.

1. Model healthy conflict behaviors and communication skills.

2. Listen and ask open-ended questions.

3. Resist participating in negative talk.[39] Redirect the conversation to address behaviors and solutions.

4. Share perspectives that defuse and reframe conflict as opportunity.

5. Support others with encouragement and teaching.

6. Encourage mediation assistance if conflict is heated and stuck. Mediators offer direction without taking on the resolution work.[40]

One of the most powerful perceptions we can bring to conflict is the potential for reconciliation. We need to believe in the possibility of harmony in order to help others see and hear new possibilities in their journeys.

Voices from the Field: Promote kindness and respect.

"Organizational cultures can become negative with a lot of conflict, yelling, and harsh treatment. Leaders need to intentionally create an environment where core values are lived out. Everyone has a role promoting kindness and respect." Douglas, Veterinarian, Canada

---

Allow New Possibilities to Move Forward

Reconciliation goes beyond resolution to invite new possibilities.[41] Corrie ten Boom, a Holocaust survivor, described the power of reconciliation she experienced in an interaction with a former SS guard who heard her speak about forgiveness after World War II. When he thanked her for the powerful message and held out his hand to shake hers, she was overwhelmed by a flood of memories.

She could see the armed guards mocking her, piles of discarded clothing, and her sister Betsy's pale face. Once again, she felt the vivid pain of Betsy's death. Corrie couldn't shake his hand until she prayed for the ability to forgive. She wrote, "As I took his hand, the most incredible thing happened. From my shoulder along my arm and through my hand a current seemed to pass from me to him, while into my heart sprang a love for this stranger that almost overwhelmed me."[42]

The reconciliation Corrie ten Boom experienced brought healing and a way to move forward. It did not include acceptance of what happened.[43] Reconciliation doesn't suggest a token apology and continuation of a hurtful environment. Rather, it provides a new path landscaped with forgiveness, peace, and hope.[44] Desmond and Mpho Tutu observed, "Forgiveness opens the door to peace between people and opens the space for peace within each person."[45]

As much as we may want to pursue reconciliation, some people simply aren't able to or aren't interested in doing so. When this happens, we are left to pick up the pieces by processing what happened and moving on our own path with forgiveness. Conflict is a part of life, but it does not need to be the primary force determining where your path goes and what it looks like.

A journey with unresolved conflict often includes loss—another life reality that rattles our world. We experience loss at a variety of levels, and it almost always changes the scenery. We will now turn toward healing from losses and helping others do so as well. Even when conflict and loss hit without warning, we can move forward with resilience.

GUIDE TO THRIVE STRATEGIES

1. Foster a perspective of conflict as a natural part of life that can reveal important truths and bring about positive changes.

2. Identify unhelpful conflict behaviors you tend to use, and replace them with healthy responses.

3. Deal with conflict in ways that reflect important values, virtues, and purpose.

4. Use conflict strategies.

5. Manage time as an ally.

6. Make use of thoughtful strategies to navigate difficult conflict situations involving power differences or highly emotional individuals.

7. Help others deal with conflict without taking on their responsibility.

8. Promote openness toward reconciliation.

Discussion Questions

How does conflict affect your role?

What makes disagreements hard to handle?

How can you make conflict seem less threatening and more transformational?

What are some positive examples of conflict resolution?

How can you help your family or team deal with conflict in healthier ways?

Would you like to discuss any other concepts or skills from the chapter?

Chapter 7

RECOVER FROM LOSS

*We can help ourselves and others find a way
to journey with hope after loss.*

Carry Hope

Loss, like conflict, creates clouds that make it harder to see beauty along the caregiver journey. Hope may seem to disappear when we feel powerless to change circumstances, but we can hold that light out for each other. Lisa, a firefighter, struggled with a mix of tragedy and helplessness as she looked upon the infant she and her team tried to revive.

The baby wore the same soft one-piece pajamas Lisa sometimes dressed her baby in. With lights flashing and sirens blaring, she and her team had rushed to the home after receiving an emergency call from the panic-stricken mother. Her baby would not wake up. Lisa tearfully held the grief-stricken mother when it was clear they could not revive her baby.

As the crew solemnly drove back to the station, Lisa was overwhelmed with questions. "Why did I, a new mother, need to be at such a traumatic call?" She thought, "What if I had to endure such loss?" Questions persisted as Lisa went home and gazed upon her smiling, kicking infant.

A year later, Lisa and her team responded to a triggered smoke alarm at the same home. As soon as the mother saw her, she gave Lisa a big hug. She thanked Lisa for her support on the day her baby died. "Everything became clear," Lisa said, "That woman needed another mom to hold her and cry with her in her deepest grief. I could not change the fact her child had died, but I could help her find comfort in knowing she wasn't alone."

We, like Lisa, can hold out the light of hope amid grief, even when we can't see it ourselves at times of loss. The life-changing losses we witness and endure mark our journey in unpredictable ways, yet we can find strength and healing. What losses have altered your world? Just as important, what has resilience looked like afterward? I know how life changing grief journeys can be after decades of walking with people enduring loss and experiencing my own.

Deaths of beloved people and animals often are the first losses we remember. However, we may experience a wide variety of life-altering losses, such as the end of a relationship, retirement from a career, or changes in health. Witnessing other people's trauma can lead to a loss of ideals, safety, and trust. No doubt about it—loss hurts. We can't erase the pain, but we can recover from loss while holding hands with others during their difficult times.

Times of walking with others in the midst of grief can be overwhelming, but also profoundly meaningful. Shannon, a veterinarian, noted, "We often deal with death. One day I helped six families face the loss of their pets. It can take a toll, but it is a blessing to be there for animals and people during hard times." The toll becomes heavier when our own grief adds to the complexity of helping others deal with loss.

Loss affects life's scenery as it changes realities, goals, hopes, roles, and dreams. How we handle grief directly affects role sustainability. Let's look at ways to help ourselves and others recover from loss. We will consider resilience and the grief process, as well as how culture influences healing. We may not be able to erase the difficult colors of grief, but we can learn to see the vibrant shades of hope in the mix.

///

Resilience at Work: Imagine . . .

Your world has shifted. A loss has touched you deeply. Grief is magnified by an emotional reexperiencing of past losses. As hard as this is, you know there will be a new normal where hope grows. You acknowledge the roller coaster of emotions and compassionately embrace yourself. Support from others holds you up when it is difficult to stand on your own. Even though life looks different, you see a new path with renewed strength and purpose.

///

Move Beyond Unhealthy Cultural Norms

Culture influences every part of life, including how we experience loss. Sometimes we need to move past unhealthy cultural norms to foster healing. I witnessed this while officiating at the memorial service for a motorcycle gang leader. After parking my blue minivan amid a sea of motorcycles, I inched my way through the crowded funeral home.

Hundreds of tough-looking motorcyclists dressed in black leather and chains gathered to honor a friend who had tragically died. Most wore red bandannas on their heads and had patches on their jackets saying things like "F*** You!" Despite their tough exterior, people from various gangs hugged, cried, and expressed caring words.

During the service, a gang leader, who towered next to me, lovingly spoke about his friend. Before finishing, this hardened man wept. I gently set my hand on his shoulder, and he gave me a big hug. Tough guys do cry, and there is no shame in this. The memorial service shattered a variety of cultural assumptions and stereotypes.

Social walls separating groups disappeared to allow mutual respect, care, and emotional expression. We can provide authentic, caring support in our shared human expression of grief whatever culture we live and work in. How we understand grief is influenced, but should not be confined, by organizational or social cultural norms.

Culture is a powerful force that includes unwritten rules about what is and is not appropriate.[1] It consists of assumptions about the correct way to think, perceive, feel, and deal with challenges.[2] Cultures valuing elders, past generations, and the natural world provide meaningful ways of honoring life and processing grief. Societal and organizational cultures that shame emotional expression make grief more complicated. When culture harms rather than helps, we can go beyond stereotypes and norms that get in the way of healing.

Voices from the Field: Go beyond unhealthy expectations.

"During a good share of my career, I was trying to figure out who I had to be as a firefighter. I tend to express emotions more easily, but early role models worked with the attitude that you had to be tough and not show emotions. Later in my career, I was able to be myself, and that felt good." Mark, Firefighter, United States

Leaders play an important role in encouraging team members to process grief when cultural norms get in the way. Charles, a paramedic, explained, "We are human beings. Responding to humans in crisis is going to affect us. Giving responders an opportunity to share after traumatic events helps tremendously. Leaders who allow people to share their emotions show care and create a more sustainable environment."

If you are in a culture that inhibits expressions of grief, find people you can safely share with. Develop a basic understanding of typical grief responses to promote acceptance and resilience. We may have to live with the powerful force of culture, but we also can face the pieces of grief honestly to promote healing and resilience.

Voices from the Field: Face loss with dignity.

"In Native American culture, there is a great connection with animals. We all are a part of the circle of life. Death is part of this circle. When I do hospice work, I am a veterinarian, social worker, and spiritual presence. It is an honor to be with people and animals at the time of death. We need to spend more time helping people and animals face the end of life with dignity and then celebrate their life after they have died." Raye, Veterinarian, United States

Connect Resilience with Pieces of Grief

Resilience and grief work together to help us recover from loss.[3] Steve and I experienced this when his mother died. Ruth made the best homemade bread. After smelling its rich aroma fill the house, I loved having a piece when it was still warm.

Alzheimer's steadily changed what my smart, capable mother-in-law could do. It was heartbreaking when she couldn't remember how to turn the oven on or call us by name. After years of saying goodbye to the person we knew, Ruth died. Anticipating her death was a grief process all on its own, but after saying goodbye for the final time, we still had to travel grief's difficult path.[4] We experienced the emotional roller-coaster ride, oscillating between happy remembrances, sadness, and other pieces of grief.

Grief is the natural process we go through to heal and accept life's new reality after loss.[5] It moves us to let go of the past, remember with love rather than pain, and work toward building a new future.[6] How we experience loss is as individualistic as the path we walk on.[7] No typical timeline, sequence, or experience is needed for healing. Some people experience intense reactions, whereas others encounter a more gradual recovery.

The journey of grief usually involves oscillating between emotions.[8] We deep dive into pain at times and then have moments when we lighten up to reconnect with the world. Lighter moments don't diminish the depth of loss, but they give us relief and make bereavement more tolerable. We can let go of preconceived notions of how we should feel after a loss and embrace resilient moments that provide glimpses of hope.

"Grief is like a long valley," C.S. Lewis explained, "a winding valley where any bend may reveal a totally new landscape."[9] The recovery process is unpredictable, but it may include certain elements typically experienced after loss.[10] As strange as it may sound, pieces of grief such as the emotional mix, bargaining, remembering, and acceptance help us find resilience and move toward a new future.

Emotional mix: The grief process includes a variety of emotions. Initially there may be shock and numbness when a loss is too difficult to process all at once.[11] Denial peeks in during moments of expecting to see a loved one walk through the door or hoping to wake up from a bad dream. Movement in and out of denial is nature's way of letting in as much as we can handle.

Like denial, anger helps us get ready to handle emotions more difficult to process. Anger associated with loss does not always make sense, but often appears because we have more experience regulating it.[12] Sometimes the anger we feel is simply a ledge to stand on after the initial free fall from loss and doesn't have a greater reason behind it.[13]

Denial and anger often give way to sadness, guilt, and loneliness. As difficult as it can be, sadness means we connected meaningfully to whom or what we lost. Heartache can feel overwhelming but will fluctuate and decrease over time.[14] Sadness becomes more complicated when feelings of guilt and loneliness are part of the landscape. We may experience guilt even if nothing could have been done differently, and loneliness can appear while being surrounded by others.[15]

Emotions of all shades turn our attention inward so we can reflect more deeply, provide self-care, and adjust to a different life.[16] This important work of moving through grief helps us find and build resilience. Moments of hope, gratitude, and happiness provide opportunities of reprieve from the heavy work as well as glimpses of healing after loss.

Voices from the Field: Allow feelings.

"When a patient who struggled with depression committed suicide, I had a strong feeling I should have done something different. Even though I did everything I could, I still felt there was something I should have done to prevent it. The family also struggled with this. I needed to join them in the 'should have' space of feeling guilty and sad." Faris, Physician, United States

---

Bargaining: It is natural to want life to return to the way it was before, so it isn't surprising that bargaining is part of grief. Even when we know the loss is final, we still may try to make deals with ourselves,

God, or others. Bargains such as "If I live differently, can I wake up from this bad dream?" or "If I do something good, then I won't lose anyone else" can provide a reprieve from the intense pain and help us move toward different pieces of grief.[17]

Remembering: Sharing stories and memories is especially healing.[18] Tears will be part of this, but so will smiles. Allow yourself to laugh and joyfully remember when moved to do so. Moments of joy don't remove all of the pain, but do remind us the sadness won't last forever. Remembering moves us to think about how our life was touched by those we lost and how the relationships continue to shape our journey.

Acceptance: We recognize the reality and permanence of our loss as healing occurs.[19] This does not mean we're okay with what happened, but it does indicate we accept that our world has changed. We realize we don't need to let go of who we are, we just need to adapt to a new future. Acceptance is not an end stage, but flickers in and out until firmly settling into a new norm.[20] Coming to terms does not diminish a loss; rather, it involves bringing the loss's meaning forward so we can invest in future plans, goals, and relationships.

> *With each and every loss comes the potential for change, growth, new insights, understanding, and refinement—all positive descriptions and words of hope. But they are often in the future, and we fail to see that far ahead when we are in the midst of our grief.* — H. Norman Wright

As difficult as loss can be, resilience is the norm, not the exception.[21] However, for some people grief interferes with functioning for several years or longer or is so intense it is self-destructive. When this happens, mental health-care providers play an important role in helping us move forward on life's journey. Getting help for the road to recovery reveals strength and wisdom, not weakness.

Recovery from loss is not a one-time conclusion, but a process.[22] When we experience new losses, it is normal for past losses to compound the grief. We don't just get over significant losses—they become a part of our journey. Resilience doesn't mean developing a life without sorrow, but regaining an ability to promote healing and thrive with the changes we carry.

Promote Healing

We can invite healing into the grief process proactively. I couldn't remove the sadness after Toivo, my daughter's beloved dog, died, but I could promote recovery. Cancer aggressively consumed our happy five-year-old, stick-chasing yellow Labrador. After he died, I made a book filled with pictures and Toivo lessons, including these:

- Life is a gift. Find joy. Smile and wag your tail even when it's hard.

- Appreciate simple pleasures.

- Life is not just about the destination. Enjoy the journey.

- Respect yourself. Respect others. Respect the world.

- Love so well that when you are gone, those you loved know how to love better.

- Remember: there's always hope.

Sophie, Steve, and I laughed, hugged, and cried as we looked at the pictures . . . Toivo photo-bombing Sophie's graduation pictures and eating ice cream on the beach. We shared stories about Toivo watching out the window and kissing Sophie every time she returned home. We gave thanks for his presence in our lives and for each other. Making the book and sharing memories was therapeutic.

We cannot remove the pain of loss, but we can help ourselves and others move toward recovery. Time spent on healing activities promotes resilience and role sustainability. As you look at the following suggestions, keep in mind cultural influences and traditions. What will help you navigate through grief and help others do so as well?

Provide self-care: Eat a hot meal, take a bath, or go on a walk. Care of basic needs increases our strength and resilience to deal with grief's demands.[23] Include opportunities for self-compassion and give yourself a hug. Adding to our suffering does not increase the significance of a loss, but instead makes it harder to honor that loss.[24] Self-care is not selfish—it's a must.

Express and communicate: Cry, talk to a friend, meet with a grief counselor, and write in a journal. Expressing emotions, thoughts, and memories is one of the best ways to promote recovery. Sharing grief with others deepens our relationships. Giving voice to memories and feelings helps us make sense of what we have a hard time grasping and enables us to remember what is important.[25]

Allow yourself to experience happy, hopeful moments: Laugh when you remember something funny. There are a lot of hard emotions, so it's important to allow lighter times. Bits of hope and happiness help us to do the hard work of grief and realize the future has possibilities.[26] They help us shift from negative to positive thought patterns.[27] How we experience life after a loved one dies is not only a testament to how they touched our lives, but also an indicator of how we honor their presence on the continuing journey.

Draw from faith: Meditate, pray, read inspirational writings, and spend time with people who provide spiritual encouragement. Faith in a divine presence means being open to what we don't understand and letting go of the need to control. It opens the door to possibilities of sacred connections and life beyond. Moments when the extraordinary touches the ordinary provide hope and help us let go of questions we may never have answers for.

Losses rattle our world and force us to reconstruct how we understand life, so it is not surprising that questioning faith might be part of the process. God can handle our doubt and anger. You are a beloved child of God—nothing within or beyond the world can change this.

Ask for help: Talk with a counselor, allow someone to pick up groceries, or have family members take the children on outings. Any time is the right time to ask for help. Assistance helps us get through the overwhelming fatigue grief causes.[28] If you are hesitant to receive help, think about how you would respond if someone asked you for support. As a caregiver, you know it is a blessing to be able to support others. It is also a blessing to receive care.

Voices from the Field: Ask for help.

"It is hard when you can't help people because they don't let you know they need help. I have had three colleagues and friends take their own lives. There was a lot of cumulative trauma, and they didn't share their suffering. I try to give support when and wherever I can, but it's also up to other people and how they respond. I want to let people know they can ask for help. People do care about them." Allen, Firefighter and Paramedic, United States and International

---

Forgive: Let go of anger and guilt by throwing a stone into a lake or giving yourself a hug. One of the most freeing things we can do is to forgive. This may include forgiving yourself, the one who has died, or others. Guilt can be a dangerous distraction from the pain of loss, so if you can't shake it loose, talk with someone who can help.[29] Forgiveness is the wind that can put us back on course.

Participate in meaningful rituals: Hold a memorial service, go to a special place, or plant a tree in honor of someone. Rituals and traditions provide strength through opportunities to observe, remember, and structure beliefs.[30] They bring people together to honor the deceased, share memories, and remind us we are not alone. Be creative and keep rituals simple. Meaningful rituals help us appreciate the past, honor the present, and look toward the future.

Intentionally care for yourself to promote healing after experiencing life-changing loss. We can help others more effectively when self-care is part of our own lives. The wounds we carry from loss don't have to stop us in our tracks. With healthy perspective and strategies, we can find strength to help others in the midst of their loss.

RECONNECT WITH YOURSELF

Important values, virtues, and purpose relate to the core of who you are outside of any relationship or role. Spend time reconnecting with this important part of who you are when you're struggling with personal loss or exposure to someone else's loss.

- Look at your purpose statement, values, and virtues.

- Write a piece of your history or make a picture collage.

- Articulate how loved ones helped you discover more about yourself. We bring people's spirit into the world as we honor the ways they positively shaped us.

- Mindfully acknowledge emotions and respond with self-compassion.

- Remember healthy limits and give yourself permission to let go of what isn't yours to carry.

As we begin to see beyond loss, we find energy to reinvest in the purpose and goals nourishing our continued journey.

Voices from the Field: Be a kind presence.

"Many times, when I have been with patients, they share great sadness with me. Perhaps they just lost someone they loved or had something else very difficult happen. I have to give psychological first aid. I want to help them more, but it's so hard because I can't do much. I just try to be a kind presence for them." Marlon, Dentist, Honduras

Help Others Recover from Loss

We cannot remove grief, but we can help others process loss. Teams, like individuals, benefit from opportunities for remembrance after a shared loss. I led a sharing time for our staff after Roger, a long-time and beloved colleague, died. Roger loved Little Debbie snacks, so I began our time of remembrance by passing one to each person. While munching the treats, we shared memories about how Roger hid candy in the clinic drawers, joked with staff, and compassionately cared for terminally ill animals and their people.

Laughter, tears, and expressions of gratitude filled our brief time remembering a dear person who touched so many lives. Roger was a good friend, so my own grief was present as I helped the team share and process their loss. My own tears and smiles mingled with everyone else's.

We can be a stabilizing force for others without denying our own emotions.[31] We just need to learn how to carry our experience while helping others. Some ways to promote healthy helping include remembering together, maintaining a sense of self, understanding grief, asking and listening, gracefully helping, and increasing cultural awareness. A variety of strategies enables us to support others without taking on their grief as well.

Remember together: Moments of group care are always more helpful than pretending nothing happened, because they show that each person is valued. Leading a time of remembrance doesn't require expertise, just the ability to guide conversation. Begin by acknowledging the individual and how they contributed to the team. Ask others to share memories and ways the person touched their life. You can close the time with a moment of silence, a prayer, or having people say something they appreciated about the individual.

Voices from the Field: See the meaning.

"It is a grace to be allowed into people's lives during times of deep loss and at end of life. Someone trusts you that much to allow you into such a sacred time." Debbie, Nurse, United States

---

Maintain emotional differentiation: Practice compassion, but refrain from taking on other people's journeys. Differentiation allows us to remain a calm presence at difficult times and allows others to experience their own emotional journeys.[32] When in helping roles, it is important to nurture mindfulness and self-regulation so our care is truly about helping others, not about ourselves.

Promote grief awareness: Reassurance about typical grief responses can help people know they are not losing touch with reality, nor are they alone in dealing with the unsettling aspects of grief.[33] For example, Amy shared that she kept expecting to see her husband, Ron, come through the door after he died. She said, "I think I am going crazy." I explained that this was a normal part of grief and she was not losing her mind.

Ask and listen: Most people find it helpful to talk about their loss, so don't be afraid to ask questions.[34] People will let you know if they are not able to talk at that moment. We process by repeating, so allow others to share their experience more than once. Let go of a need to offer solutions or anecdotes. Nothing can magically take away grief, and sometimes we just need to be silent.[35] It is hard to see people sad, but minimizing their suffering points more to our own discomfort than their needs. This is a time to simply be a calm, caring presence.

> *The friend who can be silent with us in a moment of despair or confusion, who can stay with us in an hour of grief and bereavement, who can tolerate not knowing ... not healing, not curing ... that is a friend who cares.* —Henri Nouwen

Help gracefully: Offer to help in simple ways, because even the most basic tasks can become difficult during grief.[36] Remind people to take care of basic needs so they feel empowered to put energy toward self-care. Keep in mind that grief affects every piece of life, including communication and decision-making.[37] Grieving individuals may not remember to say "Thank you" or have the energy to call you back, so be gracious and gentle.

Individual and group loss triggers many things, including the opportunity to be mindful of what we do have. Before officiating at their loved one's memorial service, I ask families what theme they would like to have, and they always say, "Celebration."

Celebrate Life Together

Even at times of loss, we can find ways to celebrate the lives of those who have died and the life we have yet to experience. Chinese New Year traditions provide a wonderful example. Lin warmly remembers carefully writing names in the family diagram posted on the wall. Special foods were set out, candles lit, and disagreements set aside for the ceremony inviting ancestors to bless family members. People are remembered, their influence is honored, and their spiritual presence acknowledged. We honor life when we bridge the past, present, and future.

Voices from the Field: Celebrate past, present, and future.

"I am inspired by my family's past and try to pass this on to my children." Lin, Family Caregiver and Educator, China and United States

---

Celebrating life together gives hope and reminds us of what is important. We remember the influence of those we have lost and become more attentive to what we have. Gratitude and other positive practices help us to find greater perspective and face loss with resilience.[38] Light does shine on the horizon, even when grief gets in the way. Sometimes we just need others to help us see hope, and other times we hold that light out for other people.

As we walk amid our own loss and the grief of others, it's okay to shed tears and ask haunting questions. However, we also need to allow ourselves to appreciate life's beauty. We can't remove loss and death as a reality in our world, but we can help others without getting swallowed up by suffering.

Our own journey is a precious gift. We can experience the radiant colors of life, especially when touched by the hues of a difficult world. Now that we have looked at how to recover from loss, we turn to the next step in the resilient and sustainable caring journey by looking at the resources that can help us thrive.

We often have more sources of support than we realize. When we reframe our definition of success to include personal wellness, we open the door to seeing and benefiting from those resources. Let's continue our resilient, sustainable journey as we unlock even more strength and reach another level of self-care, increasing our ability to thrive while helping others.

GUIDE TO THRIVE STRATEGIES

1. Understand the connections between grief, resilience, and hope.
2. Consider and move past unhealthy cultural norms connected with grief.
3. Gain a basic understanding of the process and pieces of grief.
4. Promote recovery with healing strategies.
5. Seek, as well as provide, help.
6. Use strategies to help others without taking on their grief.
7. Help teams process loss with integrity and practicality.
8. Find meaningful ways to celebrate life.

Discussion Questions

How does loss affect your helping role?

What insights do you have regarding loss and cultural norms?

How can you help yourself process grief in healthy ways?

What has it been like being with and helping people in the midst of grief?

How can you sustainably help others deal with loss?

Would you like to discuss any other ideas from the chapter?

Chapter 8

LIGHTEN THE LOAD WITH RESOURCES

We don't need to struggle alone.
We can use resources to promote vibrant caring.

See Success Differently

We want to show the world we are strong enough, talented enough, to glide gracefully through any challenge thrown at us. I get it, because I easily fall into believing I need to be self-sufficient and silent about vulnerabilities. One occasion illustrating this occurred a few days after my daughter was born. Steve had returned to work, so I was left to solo parent our new baby and preschool-aged sons.

On that pleasant summer afternoon, I took the children for a walk that ended with the cries of a hungry baby and a three-year-old temper tantrum. Upon our return home, Steve calmly met us at the door. I'm sure he could hear us a block away, and if I had paid attention, I would have noticed he was trying to communicate something important. With frustration, I thrust the baby into his arms and yelled a few things, including, "I can't handle it anymore!"

After angrily expressing myself, I finally listened to Steve. He informed us that Clyde and Helvea, members of a church I was pastor for at the time, were sitting in the living room with baby gifts. My sons and I fell deathly silent. According to my memory, even newborn Sophie became quiet.

We dusted ourselves off and walked into the living room with smiles. Helvea sheepishly commented, "This seems like a bad time to visit." I responded, "Not at all. This is great. Everything is wonderful." What a ridiculous thing to pretend perfection after they had witnessed our meltdown.

The inability to use resources and share vulnerabilities leads us down a path of suffering with little hope of change. There are a lot of reasons we have difficulty admitting that life can be hard, but wouldn't it be grand if we could be more transparent about our vulnerabilities and help others share theirs as well?

Think of the common support we could provide and receive if we talked about challenges without fear of being judged. As we drop the pretense of shouting "Look at me—I am strong enough and capable enough to help others without ever needing help," we can be more authentic and allow ourselves to use resources. This may seem easy, but getting to such authenticity often involves seeing success differently.

Resources are assets if we see them as a part of success and allow them to lighten the load. The next step of the resilient and sustainable caring journey focuses on building support. We will identify resources and consider how to overcome silencers making it hard to use them. Awareness of what makes support safe is helpful for finding resources and becoming a valuable resource for others. We also will consider how resources can help us untangle ethical dilemmas and discern when change is needed. Let's look at the abundance of resources and care that can help us thrive.

Resilience at Work: Imagine . . .

You provided help in a dire situation. Your journey has covered a lot of ground, and this certainly was not the first difficult event, but something hit you hard. Although heavy feelings create a sense of loneliness, you know you are not alone. You name challenges and face them with strength by using resources. Authentic sharing overcomes vulnerability. In the midst of difficulties, you find peace and enjoy moments that make you smile.

Know and Use Resources

We can get so focused on what's in front of us that we miss the abundance of available resources. Imagine facing a giant redwood tree in the middle of a forest. I recently stood with toes to trunk, admiring one of nature's giants. A Northern California redwood tree can soar into the sky higher than a twenty-four-story building and have a trunk wider than four refrigerators.[1] As I stared at the tree, I couldn't see the rest of the beauty surrounding me.

I continued the uphill hike to a plateau, where I looked down upon the forest. I had a much different perspective. I could see hundreds of grand redwood trees and other plants in that beautiful ecosystem. We need to step away from the tree trunk, as entrancing as it can be, to see more of the beauty.

Similar to standing before the trunk of a large tree, we can get stuck looking at a small number of resources when there is a whole forest to draw from. A resource is anything that can help us function in healthy, effective ways. But we can use the abundant supply of resources to promote sustainable caring and resilience only when we see them.

Voices from the Field: Use resources.

"Helping people is very rewarding, but it is stressful as well. Having tools to handle the stress is important. Talking with others whom you feel safe sharing with can help you process the stressful challenges and understand how to deal with them." Kris, Physician, United States

---

Technical websites, mentors, and professional groups are among the resources we first think of when it comes to professional roles. Mentors and colleague groups can provide great perspective, especially when we invest in such relationships.[2] Caregivers in other disciplines also can offer important insights. Support sources extend far beyond the context of any single helping role.

Family members, a book group, a nearby park, or a beloved pet are important on any resource list. Professionals such as counselors, clergy, coaches, and spiritual directors can help us see situations differently while providing encouragement. Accessing professional help before we hit crisis stage prevents secondary trauma and leads to more effective processing when life gets hard.[3]

Add freely to your resource list. Name individuals rather than clumping them in a group. For example, I could list "family" as a resource, or I could name Steve, Josh, Caleb, Sophie, and others to denote more adequately people I can turn to for help. Your resource list should help you see the abundance of support available, especially when life is hard.

Toivo, Karma, and Mindy are dogs that provided great support to me with their calm, gentle presence during challenges. Research confirms what most of us have known for years: animals can help us decrease stress, recover from trauma, and improve well-being.[4] One study indicates having a dog can reduce self-judgment and increase self-compassion.[5] It's hard not to smile and feel nourished when a furry friend expresses joy simply because you are with it.

Be creative as you think about what nourishes you. Important resources also include fitness activities and relaxing or creative pastimes. Hike with friends, paint a picture, or read a novel. Name places where you find peace and energy. Perhaps a path through the woods or a lake's shoreline. We are made to be in connection with the world around us, so time with nature can be among the most nourishing. See the forest rather than staring at a trunk when it comes to resources.

BRAINSTORM RESOURCES

Write down what you see as available resources. Once you think you have a good list, be creative, think harder, and expand your list to at least thirty resources. Consider those that you may take for granted. Recognize as many sources of support as possible, and then foster a willingness to use them.

Once you have a list, consider how you use resources. If you have difficulty using certain resources, think about why and how you can change your hesitancy. Give yourself permission to use all of your resources to lighten the load.

We find comfort knowing we have many sources of support to draw from, but we need to allow ourselves to use those resources. Insights and encouragement from a variety of sources promote a sustainability and healing we can't develop on our own. [6] If you are reluctant to ask for help, consider why. We can come up with a multitude of excuses for not using resources, but they usually aren't good reasons.

Failure to use resources makes the journey harder, turning gentle hills into treacherous mountains. Or worse yet, we get stuck looking at just one tree trunk in the forest. But sometimes we need to confront silencers before we can move forward and see more.

Voices from the Field: Let's be authentic.

"I used to be more stoic and afraid to show how I am feeling. Now, after many years, I am more likely to tear up and express emotion. I am more authentic. I feel more like myself . . . It is critical to have a shared community, people you can talk to, especially when struggling. It is so easy to feel isolated and beat up on yourself if you don't." Mike, Veterinarian, United States

---

Overcome Silencers

As you consider using resources, do any of the following come to mind?

- I don't have time or energy.
- No one else seems to need help.
- I don't want to be a bother.
- I am the only one who struggles.
- Others will think I am weak.
- I need to succeed on my own.

You are not alone if such thoughts disrupt your use of resources. They are effective silencers springing from a variety of sources and perceptions. Silencers prevent us from reaching out for help and speaking authentically with others.

We do need to be selective regarding when, where, and with whom to share. However, talking about difficult experiences promotes well-being.[7] Sometimes we diminish our own needs or get caught up in unrealistic expectations. We seldom hear about other people's vulnerabilities, so we mistakenly believe we are the only ones struggling. Such perceptions make it hard to promote self-care and authenticity. Remaining true to ourselves is always more sustainable than pretending to be someone different.

"Authenticity is the daily practice of letting go of who we think we're supposed to be and embracing who we are," explained Brené Brown.[8] This involves facing unrealistic expectations, including perfectionism. As we noted earlier, perfectionism and shame often travel together and are among the most effective silencers we need to overcome.

Voices from the Field: Remember others struggle also.

"When I learned other people struggle with the same things I did, I felt understood. Like I wasn't alone. After this, I felt more free and less guilty to take a break and do things to take care of myself. Then I could help more." Rommel, Nonprofit Leader and Volunteer, Honduras

---

Shame screams some of the most dangerous messages, such as "You don't belong."[9] It creates a fear of sharing vulnerabilities and pushes us toward isolation. Ironically, our need for connection with others becomes the focus, while we get sidelined by fears of rejection. We move away from purpose-driven living and have difficulty honoring healthy limits.[10] We close the door to deeper care and sustainability, rather than share vulnerabilities.

Marlon, a dentist in Honduras, was so burned out he couldn't go to the office. Shame had closed and locked the door to authentic sharing. He explained, "The work and need never stop. I didn't talk about my struggles, because people see being vulnerable as a sign of weakness. A friend who cared enough encouraged me to find help. I began to heal when I could talk about what was hard. We are all human and vulnerable at times."

> "Wholeness does not mean perfection; it means embracing brokenness as an integral part of life" —Parker Palmer[11]

We don't have to struggle alone, but it is too easy to put walls around our hearts when we expect too much or feel the weight of other people's expectations. The more we live with walls in one part of life, the harder it is to dismantle them in other contexts. One of the best things we can do is embrace our own humanity and allow ourselves to talk with others.

Helpful sharing moves us toward healing and positivity.[12] This doesn't mean getting stuck in a complaint and negativity mode. Paired with self-compassion, talking about vulnerabilities helps us loosen the grip of unrealistic expectations and include wellbeing in our definition of success.[13]

Connections with others provide a wonderful array of resources, especially when we overcome silencers to authentically share. We open doors to meaningful connections as we live from core principles and purpose, rather than fears and negativity.[14] Reliable relationships help us bounce back from challenges and provide a safe haven when we feel vulnerable.[15]

DEFINE SUCCESS TO INCLUDE WELL-BEING

What does success look like to you? Write down what you see as successful in your helping role. Ideally, your important values, virtues, and purpose fit right into this definition.

Expand your idea of achievement to include personal well-being, healthy relationships, and the use of resources. Consider the importance of resilience and sustainability. Go ahead, maintain high standards, but let go of perfectionism.

Now what does success look like? Redefine success to embrace your humanness and all of life's journey.

Promote Safe Support

Think about someone who has been a safe source of support for you. What was different about them? How did they help you feel comfortable enough to share? Safe, supportive relationships are truly a gift. Social support is critical in preventing and healing from challenges such as compassion fatigue.[16] Unfortunately, reliable connections seem to be a rare blessing in our complicated world.

Voices from the Field: Find and provide safe support.

"Being able to talk about hard things with others is so helpful. Early in my career, I had a strong mentorship with a boss I respected, which was so important. I could talk about my vulnerabilities without being ashamed. Now I try to be someone others can share with." Lauren, Veterinarian, United States

We all have history with relationship challenges. Our paths are littered with broken connections we thought were going to fill life with joy forever. The lingering effects of such experiences can make it hard to risk being vulnerable and open.[17] The following characteristics of healthy relationships can help us identify who to turn to for safe support, as well as how to offer it to others:

- Mutual respect shown through care and positive communication.

- Acceptance based on authentic connection rather than approval or achievement.[18]

- Deep listening without interruption or need to fix everything.[19]

- Grounding in common humanity so there is reciprocal sharing of vulnerabilities and challenges[20] (mutual sharing doesn't apply to connections with professional providers).

- Ability to share different perspectives without fear of judgment, blame, or shame.[21]

- Honoring of privacy and confidentiality.

- Ability to regulate emotions and differentiate experiences from those of the other person.[22]

- Interactions that promote positive perspective and hope, even with challenges.

What characteristics would you add? What can you do differently to be a safer resource for others? Relationships exhibiting such qualities rarely just happen but usually require intentional development and personal growth. Healthy relationships help us bring out the best in ourselves even in the midst of difficult dilemmas.

PRACTICE SHARING THE DIFFICULT

Rehearse talking about challenges to get past silencers. Take steps to broaden your ability to share vulnerabilities. Potential activities include the following:

- Look in the mirror and voice difficulties out loud.

- Tell your furry loved one all about something bothering you.

- Write down what is hard and have someone safe read it.

- Talk about a past challenge with a trustworthy person.

- Meet with a professional (counselor, therapist, pastor, or coach) who you know will keep what you say confidential.

- Share with one or two individuals privately.

- Request team or family meetings and include time to address topics focused on wellness.

- Raise questions among small groups of colleagues, friends, or family that invite deeper conversation.

Practice helps us become more comfortable with talking about hard things. We will often find that by sharing wisely and authentically, we encourage others to do the same.

Voices from the Field: Seek a reliable group.

"Find a group of people that can help to keep you real and provide mutual support. People you can ask, "Is this what you experienced, or is it just me?" People who are focused on doing the right thing rather than their own success." Wade, Physician, United States

Untangle Ethical Dilemmas

What dilemmas challenge your beliefs? When does your helping role bump up against your moral well-being and sense of what is right?

- Shauna, a mental health-care provider, experienced this when she saw health-care providers fail to give patients in a mental health unit the same care they gave other patients.
- Dan, a firefighter and paramedic, struggles each time his team is called to nursing homes through 911 to lift a resident off the floor and place them back in their bed,

while staff who could have helped the resident stand by and watch.

- Lauren, a veterinarian, bumps into this every time she deals with a sick animal and the owners can't or won't spend the money needed for care.

- John, a physician, experienced this as the organization increased patient load while decreasing assistants, so staff were doing tasks they weren't qualified for.

Ethical dilemmas don't announce themselves, so it can be hard to know when we are facing one.[23] If a problem keeps bothering you, chances are something is bumping up against your sense of what is right and wrong. Repeated demands to act in ways opposing personal values and morals can lead to distress, burnout, and other challenges.[24] Violation of deeply held beliefs has psychological, social, behavioral, and spiritual health repercussions.[25]

Situations involving moral problems shouldn't be easy or quick to solve, because they have many ramifications. However, it is worth taking the energy to process ethical dilemmas for a number of reasons, including personal wellness and sustainability. Ignoring them will simply add to the heaviness of helping roles. Resources, along with important values and principles, provide valuable guidance for untangling challenges with integrity.[26]

The following is a framework for processing ethical dilemmas:

1. **What?** Define the problem.

   o Be as specific, objective, and concise as possible. Your initial answer may be a symptom of a deeper systemic problem. If so, dig deeper.

2. **Why?** Note why it is important for you to deal with the issue or let it go.

   o Look at important values, virtues, and purpose, both personal and organizational. Professional and legal standards also should be considered. How other people are affected is another important factor. Feedback from objective resources can provide helpful perspective.

   o Determine whether or not to take action.

3. **How?** If you feel there is good enough reason to deal with the problem, brainstorm potential solutions and their implications.

   o Think outside of the box. Enlist help from creative thinkers to develop an array of possibilities.

   o Choose what you see as the best option. Ethical dilemmas seldom provide ideal solutions and often force a choice between difficult alternatives.

   o Get objective feedback from someone you trust outside of the group or system involved in the dilemma.

4. **When?** Choose when to act for the best possibility of a positive outcome.

   o Remember, the best time is not when emotions are running high.

   o Assess the response. Was there resolution, or do you need to try another tactic? It often takes time and repeated efforts to deal with serious problems, especially in larger organizations or systems.

We should choose our battles carefully while also honoring our moral health. Intentional processing of difficult dilemmas helps us define what we will tolerate. Guiding values, beliefs, and purpose provide the courage to promote change. Outside resources offer perspective to see situations and solutions differently.

We don't need to struggle on our own but can benefit from a variety of resources. Sometimes, we diligently work to untangle the difficult, but still can't find balance or wellness. When the difficult remains too difficult, resources can help us discern if it's time to change our role or work environment.

Know When to Change a Role

Leaving a position to sustain personal wellness can be difficult. I know how hard it is to invest energy and heart in helping others but have an organization or individuals continually challenge your efforts to promote healthy change. We envision the good we can do, but it is derailed repeatedly by negativity. I decided to leave such a position after many tears, discussions, and prayers.

The organization had more than a century of unresolved conflict and faced a serious lack of money. Leaders hired me to bring about lifesaving organizational changes. I continually faced conflict and resistance to change. Over time, I realized I was not going to be able to bring about needed changes. Just as important, the position took a serious toll on my health, despite my continued efforts to promote balance.

I wanted to run away, fast and far, but it took months to discern whether I should leave. I documented successes and challenges. I identified personal signs of imbalance, such as sleeplessness, physical pain, sadness, and hopelessness. I wrote down what I wasn't willing to give up: the joy of personal relationships, the ability to exercise, my faith in God, and a healthy belief in myself. I set a time frame of six months and dug in to turn things around using resources.

At the end of six months, I reviewed the list and assessed the situation. Despite my efforts, the environment had become less sustainable. I let go of my commitment and hopes in that difficult setting. Intentionality didn't take away the pain, but it did protect my integrity and promote healing.

Resilience is the ability to bounce back.[27] Sometimes this means recovering after leaving a difficult environment. Workplaces can become toxic, contributing to compassion fatigue and burnout.[28] Systemic negativity and cynicism make it harder for everyone to thrive. Whether it is because of organizational culture, personal circumstances, or other individuals, it can be too difficult to find balance in a role or setting. We get stuck.

Too many boundaries have been crossed or neglected to get back to a healthy place. Take immediate steps if urgency is needed for safety. Unless there is imminent danger, intentional processing of difficult situations is usually more helpful for long-term functioning than an abrupt departure.[29] How we leave a position will determine our journey afterward.

STRATEGY TO DISCERN A NEED FOR CHANGE

1. Spend time considering why change might be needed, while looking at the disadvantages and advantages of change.

2. Identify signs of personal imbalance and lack of health. Think of physical symptoms, emotional changes, social behaviors, cognitive perceptions, and spiritual lows you experience when struggling.

3. Determine what degree of imbalance you will not accept, and assess how you are doing. What are you not willing to give up? We gladly make sacrifices to help other people, but we also need to be aware of what we are not willing to lose.

4. Remember important values and purpose. Consider whether you can honor them in the current context.

5. Determine how much longer you will try to establish healthy balance in the role. If your well-being has not improved by that date, give yourself permission to let go.

6. Use resources. Because our perceptions can become cloudy or skewed when struggling, feedback from professionals and safe people can help us navigate the dense emotions and remind us what is healthy.[30]

If you believe it is time to change a role or working environment, create a strategy so you can leave in a way that decreases personal and organizational trauma. Unfortunately, how we exit a situation can have a bigger impact than the good work we did. Change or leave a position with your integrity intact, and you will be able to find a healthy balance much sooner. A role change doesn't mean our helping journey comes to an end—it just takes on different scenery.

DEVELOP A PLAN FOR CHANGE

1. Create a timeline for when you will communicate intentions and leave or change your role. If able, include personal time for processing and healing afterward.

2. Describe how you will leave. Be specific about personal attitude and behavior. Clarify what and how you hope to communicate. Remember the presence you strive to bring into the world, and commit to reflecting your important values, virtues, and purpose.

3. Plan what you will do after leaving. Address needs and create possibilities to look forward to that promote healing.

4. List resources and how you will use them in the process.

Be Your Best Resource

Our helping journey continues to shape the world with care even after significant changes. We are never alone in bringing care to others in times of life challenges and trauma. An abundance of resources is available to guide and support. Wherever we are on our journey of helping others, our resources can change and expand—possibilities are unlimited.

The most important resource you have for promoting resilience and sustainability is—you. You are the one who can define success in a way that includes your own well-being. You decide what resources to develop and use to lighten the load. Make a commitment to be your own best resource, and open the door to other sources of support.

Advocating for yourself and doing the work to build resilience are important for sustainability. You are worth being cared for. You are the one who can counter challenges and choose how to perceive life experiences. Other people provide important perspective, but don't deny the significance of your own knowledge when it comes to your authentic journey.

You know better than anyone else what you believe, need, and long for. You choose the direction to take, but you are never alone. In fact, even if you can't see them, many others are walking alongside you in the wonderful journey of bringing heart into the world. Don't just take my word for it, but look for people on similar paths.

Now that we have a grasp on resources, we will take the next step toward resilient, sustainable caring with ideas for growing a community of support. When we expand and rely on a supportive community, we can shine brighter than any of us ever can alone. We all benefit from and shape the groups we are part of to influence collective resilience and well-being. Are you ready to experience a deeper level of care? Let's take the next step!

GUIDE TO THRIVE STRATEGIES

1. Develop an expansive resource list.

2. Encourage yourself to use resources.

3. Reframe your definition of success to include well-being and use of resources.

4. Overcome silencers that make it hard to share authentically.

5. Practice talking about difficult topics.

6. Be open to assistance from a coach, therapist, or other helping professional.

7. Promote safe, supportive relationships.

8. Use resources to untangle ethical dilemmas.

9. Discern when a change in role or environment is needed.

10. Establish a plan for changing your role.

11. Commit to being your own best resource.

Discussion Questions

Brainstorm a list of resources. When you think you have a full list, try to come up with at least ten more items.

What do you need to do to use resources?

How do you define success to include personal well-being?

What characteristics do you see as important in supportive relationships?

How can you foster these?

Describe how you approached a difficult dilemma. What resources were helpful?

Would you handle it differently now? If so, how?

Would you like to discuss any other concepts from the chapter?

Chapter 9

GROW SUPPORTIVE COMMUNITY

We are part of something bigger than ourselves and find strength functioning as a "we" rather than a "me."

Hold Out the Light for Each Other

We can help others better by working together. The Split Rock Lighthouse provides a wonderful example of the power in working collectively. High on a rocky cliff, the lighthouse was a beacon of safety for ships crossing Lake Superior.[1] Towering pines and multicolored rocks display nature's beauty along the rugged shoreline. Storms quickly turn calm waters into nature's wrath. In 1905, a November storm damaged or sunk twenty-nine ships. That inspired the building of the bright, rotating light to guide marine traffic.

Sailors on ships carrying iron ore and grain could see the light for more than twenty-two miles from the beautiful but dangerous lakeshore. Two-hundred-and-fifty-two cut-glass prisms made up the innovative lens radiating such a powerful beacon.[2] Each piece played a role in the lighthouse's ability to help sailors navigate rough waters. Optimal effectiveness occurred only when all the pieces worked together toward the common goal of guiding ships during storms.

Like the Split Rock Lighthouse, we can radiate much more brightly together than alone. "We" is a powerful concept that involves understanding each individual is part of something bigger. Like the prisms that worked together providing a ray of hope, we can do the same for others and ourselves.

Our culture in the United States is so individualistic it is easy to forget that collectively we can prepare for, approach, and recover from difficult challenges. We can face suffering together and heal together. Ideal functioning is not individualistic, but comes from combined support and effort. Strategies to increase sustainability are most effective when they include a community of support.[3] We can help each other while changing the world together.

Even when you feel alone, more people care about you and want to support you than you realize. Plant this knowing in your core. Stubbornly counter the internal dialogue that shuts down sharing and creates feelings of isolation.[4] Remember to see the "we" of care.

We all benefit from supportive communities and play a role in making them possible.[5] Let's consider perspectives, tools, and models for developing supportive connections. We will look at ongoing groups that expand resilience and promote healing. Short-term gatherings to process trauma as a team are also important. We will touch on ways to expand your support system by changing how you see community.

I discovered the incredible value of expanding my perspective on community after decades of helping people. I truly hope it doesn't take you as long as it took me to understand the importance of supportive community for resilience and sustainable caring. As you journey on the path of helping, you hold out a light of hope for others during storms. Allow others to hold out that light for you too.

Resilience at Work: Imagine . . .

It's been a tough week, month, year. You take a calming breath and note a mix of emotions. Sadness and anger come to mind, but so do hope and satisfaction. You have stayed true to your purpose and values. After a mental hug and words of encouragement, you talk with a friend and schedule time with a coach or counselor. You know others care about you. You shed a few tears, but also smile and laugh at joyful memories. You know you are strong and, with help, will thrive. Your journey doesn't stop, but slows down to nurture healing and hope.

Build Resilience Together

We know there are going to be storms on any journey. How we process the storms will determine our ability to handle and bounce back from the challenges.[6] Groups that provide opportunities to learn, share, and support help us enjoy the journey and get through storms with grace. I have led various resilience programs, and the most influential were those involving monthly one-hour sessions.

Healthcare professionals involved in ongoing sessions found these things helpful:

- Having a safe space to share and explore fears, challenges, and struggles.

- Sharing frustrating experiences and brainstorming solutions together.

- Hearing everyone else's thoughts on a subject and realizing there is more than one way to look at something.

- Developing trust and being vulnerable with colleagues.

- Having time to discuss feelings—often one of the participants' biggest weaknesses.

- Feeling that someone cares because they want to, not because they have to.

Resilience sessions began with a guided meditation. Physicians sat around the conference-room table, some wearing scrubs and others blue jeans. Beepers and cell phones were silenced, yet managed to occasionally interrupt conversation. After the first few minutes, tapping feet and bouncing knees slowed to a stop.

The time of mindfulness helped us move on to introspective work, learning, and discussion. I introduced a concept, along with prompts for each person to reflect on. *What does living your values look like when you deal with conflict or loss? What boundaries are the hardest to maintain?* Discussions about the concepts and prompts filled the session's second half. Some participants easily talked about challenges, while others offered occasional comments.

We talked about resilience and sustainability related topics. Participants chose subjects such as how to counter compassion fatigue, deal with conflict, promote self-compassion, process loss of a colleague, and establish healthy boundaries. I offered information and practical tools. These scheduled sessions, with their mix of mindfulness, learning, and discussion, provided opportunities to talk about challenges while affirming a common ground.

A central goal was fostering a safe environment for mutual sharing. I was not a staff member, and we agreed what was said during sessions stayed within the group. Confidentiality and respect are key to any successful group. Consistent meetings increased trust and the ability to share. Over time, even those who tended to be quiet spoke more often. Some members reached out for help during difficult times. Group emphasis on self-care and growth fostered a sustainable helping environment in the organization beyond the sessions.[7]

Supportive community is essential to the prevention of compassion fatigue and other challenges.[8] Group bonding and skill building promote daily resilience while building a reservoir of strength for tougher times. Resilience, after all, is more than recovering from adversity.[9] We increase the ability to bounce back from challenges and also thrive with more wisdom and strength.

CHOOSE A SUSTAINABLE WORK ENVIRONMENT

Be proactive when it comes to choosing where and with whom you work in professional helping roles. Creating a microculture of support wherever you are is one of the best tools to increase resilience.[10] Remember, context affects sustainability.[11] Consider these strategies:

1. Keep your purpose statement, values, and virtues in mind as you consider different workplaces.[12] Location, money, and prestige certainly have pull, but role sustainability relies on much more than those factors.

2. Research an organization's purpose and values. Listen to employees' stories, look for news accounts, and examine

policies to see whether actions reflect articulated purpose and values. Make sure your purpose, values, and virtues align with the organization.[13]

3. Examine the potential for support from colleagues. Peers can provide valuable perspective and encouragement.[14] Listen to your instincts as to whether you could develop positive colleague relationships.

4. Consider mentors. Mentor relationships provide the education you didn't receive in school.[15] An ideal work environment, especially at the beginning of career, includes a mentor in the organization or community. Invest in mentor relationships and ask questions. Experienced helpers provide insights on how to deal with challenges.[16]

5. Maintain helpful connections with mentors and colleagues outside of your workplace. They can give valuable perspective without being caught up in the organization's culture.

Voices from the Field: Invest in mentor relationships.

"Mentor relationships are vital to personal and career success. Such connections are an important source of continued professional development. Cultivate positive relations with mentors through asking questions and setting goals. Having a mentor and being a mentor are rewarding personally and for the communities we work in." Douglas, Veterinarian, Canada and United States

Process Difficult Events as a Team

Helping other people is not a one-way affair, and we are called to give and receive.[17] This struck home for Mark years ago. On a sunny day, he and another firefighter found themselves dealing with a tragic accident while summer onlookers crowded around the scene. The situation seemed surreal, and the stress was intense. It was one of those experiences that stops people in their tracks and shifts life perceptions.

After the event, leaders held a critical incidence stress debriefing (CISD) session for everyone who had worked at the scene. Each participant had the opportunity to share their description of the scene, how the call came in, and what they heard, saw, or smelled. Discussion moved on to how they experienced the event, what they thought, and how they felt. Participants initially sat slouched in folding chairs with eyes glued to the floor. As people talked, they sat up straighter and looked at each other.

"I could feel and see the weight lifted off of people," explained Mark. "It felt like we had a deeper bond and could support each other better after talking about what we experienced." The CISD model provides a wonderful framework for safe sharing and mutual support. Trained peers, along with a mental health professional, lead sessions that can be requested by any participant after a traumatic event.

Developed by former first responder Jeffrey Mitchell, PhD, CISD "attempts to enhance resistance to stress reactions, build resiliency or the ability to bounce back from a traumatic experience, and facilitate both recovery from traumatic stress and a return to normal, healthy functions."[18] Critical events have the emotional power to override usual coping skills, so intervention is invaluable.[19]

Organizational leaders play a key role in promoting group sustainability through opportunities such as CISD participation. Leadership can increase team effectiveness by accepting that stressors are legitimate and that it's the organization's responsibility to promote wellness.[20] Open and effective communication about challenges at all levels normalizes adverse responses to traumas and the need for interventions. Important sharing helps us reframe and heal from adverse events.[21]

Voices from the Field: Talk about traumatic events.

"Talking about traumatic events is important. Showing vulnerability is a good way to normalize reactions to really tough things. Doing this together lets coworkers know, 'I'm trying to process this also and it isn't easy,' so we can support each other. This is much more helpful than gallows humor, dehumanizing the people we help, or ridiculing colleagues when they struggle."
Mark, Firefighter, United States

Supportive group leaders gently encourage people to share when it is difficult. Bonnie, a social worker who leads CISD sessions, recalled one occasion after a child died. The officer who had held the child sat bent over and silent almost the whole time. After being asked about the child, he hesitated, and then quietly answered, describing what happened and how he felt. Participants were deeply touched and responded with heartfelt support. Bonnie said, "Everyone was emotionally holding on to each other during this space. You could see the healing happen."

A group process to analyze difficult events can increase organizational effectiveness and employee sustainability.[22] Some health-care organizations use a peer-review process after traumatic events to analyze what happened and develop ways to improve care. Processing the difficult with others expands our perspective and reminds us we are a part of something bigger than ourselves.

We don't need to suffer alone after difficult experiences. Others can help hold up the light of hope if we feel lost, so we can get back on track more quickly. The light we radiate together doesn't just shine during the storms, but provides continued guidance for the journey. Sometimes this means recovering over the long term together.

Voices from the Field: When it gets hard, get help.

"When you are able to help someone, it's a great feeling. But dealing with traumatic times can be really tough. When it gets to be hard, get help. Talk with others, a trusted colleague, or a professional." Mike, Firefighter, United States

---

Heal with Others

We can recover from ongoing challenges by giving and receiving help from others with similar struggles.[23] Ana wholeheartedly affirms this as she talks about participation in Al-Anon meetings for thirty-five years. She explained, "I can go to an Al-Anon meeting and feel anxious or angry at everyone in the world. As the meeting begins and we read the Twelve Steps, I calm down. I see people who I know have struggled just as much as I have, and they look fine. It helps me think I can also be fine. This calms me down."

At Al-Anon, professionals, retirees, caregivers, and young adults from various economic and cultural backgrounds gather in a circle to listen and share. Some have attended hundreds of meetings, and others are there for the first time. Everyone has been negatively affected by someone's alcoholism. Meetings begin with a welcome and moment of silence ending with prayer. A leader reads the group purpose, expectations, and procedures. Who attends and what's said are kept strictly anonymous, which provides security for honest sharing.

Discussion is focused on applying the Twelve Steps to daily life. "*1. We admitted we were powerless over alcohol—that our lives had become unmanageable . . .*"[24] Participants acknowledge the common ground, have a shared goal, and understand clear guidelines. All three components help groups reach a deeper level of meaning.

Voices from the Field: Encourage others to share.

"Members have a deep connection with each other. We gather to share experiences and strengthen hope. New participants are welcomed, because we know how hard it is to be there for the first time. We all carry brokenness. We tell new group members, "You may not like everyone in the group, but you'll learn to love us." Ana, Pastor, United States

---

Lois Wilson founded Al-Anon for family members of alcoholics based on the Alcoholics Anonymous (AA) group model.[25] Al-Anon and AA have successfully helped people heal since 1935. They provide a meeting model that promotes authentic sharing, dynamic learning, and nonjudgmental support.

> *"Community does not necessarily mean living face-to-face with others; rather, it means never losing the awareness that we are connected to each other. It is about being fully open to the reality of relationship, whether or not we are alone."* —Parker Palmer[26]

Finding and developing safe spaces to promote healing requires intentional and courageous work. Sometimes we need to look outside of our surroundings and helping role to find those places. Solitary work is important for personal healing and growth, but we also need connections.[27] Our capacity for self-deception and judgment can lead us off the path, away from sustainable caring. Truly supportive people refuse to go along with harmful patterns of behavior that pull us away from a healthy journey.[28]

Healthy connections help us stay on course and bounce back higher than we could by ourselves.[29] Safe communities, characterized by trust and acceptance, allow space for the inner journey while providing a sense of accompaniment.[30] Taking the first step to connect with or lead any group can be the most difficult. Enlist the help of a safe support person to venture forward. Stepping outside of our comfort zone includes risk, but also increases community.

Voices from the Field: Have friends outside of work.

"As a leader, I couldn't go to my staff for support, so it is important to have friends outside of the organization. As colleagues in very different roles with similar goals, we could mentor each other. You need to be your own well-being police. This means making time for self-care and being with supportive people." Robyn, Youth Advocate, Honduras

Expand Understanding of Community

Our understanding of community shapes who we include in our world. My community used to be quite small, including only the people in my immediate surroundings. I discovered a whole new world of meaningful connections and support when I traveled to Honduras.

A beat-up white truck filled in the back with men and boys and clusters of barefoot children near busy streets were among my first images of Honduras. We drove by guards with machine guns on street corners and steep hillsides covered with tin shacks. I felt as though I had traveled to a different world. In some ways I had, but I have found that we have much more in common than we often think.

My world expanded with each return trip to Honduras. My support network now includes a wonderful variety of friends from Central America, Asia, and Africa. I continually learn from experiences in communities far outside of what I initially considered to be community. People with a wide array of perspectives help me see life differently and face challenges with hope. Community can be so much bigger than we think it is.

We can expand our support system by changing how we see community. David, a mental health-care provider and educator, discovered this while working at international schools in Hungary, Bangladesh, and Belgium. A walk across a campus with typical brick buildings could find students in blue jeans or a hijab—people from various continents who may say, "Hello," "Salut," or "Assalamu alaikum."

Differences are apparent, but so are similarities. David explained, "Working in international communities, we found that people focus more on commonalities rather than differences. I often talked with colleagues from around the world about the same challenges. People have very human responses and face many of the same frustrations around the world. There's more common ground than differences."

We can increase the size and depth of community by focusing on the commonalities rather than differences. Look outside your role, workplace, and living space to enjoy meaningful connections that inspire and nourish. Simple perspective changes, along with a dash of humility, can expand the possibilities of where we may find support.

Voices from the Field: Rise above biases.

"No matter how we live our lives, it always comes back to our roots. We need to rise above our own biases to provide care with a perspective of common humanity. When we bridge cultures, we open up possibilities." Rumbidzai, Family Caregiver and Sustainability Advocate, Zimbabwe and United States

How do you describe your community? Who is in it? What would a picture representing community look like for you? Now make the picture bigger—how can you expand your community?

STRATEGIES TO EXPAND YOUR COMMUNITY

- Develop awareness about how you see relationships, and then expand your perspective of who you share common ground with.[31] For example, physicians can find a lot in common with veterinarians, nurses, first responders, and other helpers. Find and offer support outside typical connections.

- Invest in relationships outside your helping role to ground yourself and increase playfulness. Play with a child, birdwatch with an elder, and walk with a friend to remember you are more than any one of your roles.

- Develop connections outside of your environment. Exploration of different cultures and social groups provides abundant opportunities for growth and nourishment.[32]

- Initiate opportunities for deeper conversations with people. Ask a colleague about an emotional case or a friend about how they find balance. They don't need to see the world exactly like you do, but just need to be willing to listen and respect your perspective.[33]

- Volunteer in settings outside of your typical environment. Spend time at the local shelter or participate in an international service trip. When we stretch the boundaries of our comfort zone, we allow more people into our understanding of community.

- Enjoy companionship with an animal. Cuddle with a kitten or walk dogs at the local shelter. The human-animal bond is powerful and can be a great source of care.
- Schedule ongoing virtual conversations with individuals you know and respect in other parts of the world.

When we expand and rely on a supportive community, we create a more helpful environment for the people we work with and for. Community and care extend far beyond the borders we often see as barriers. Perspective on the larger world helps us see connections beyond our helping roles. Supportive people with a variety of experiences offer valuable insight, especially when we are struggling. Our "together" as helpers is much bigger than we think.

Shine Brighter

Just like brilliant lighthouses providing guidance, we shine much more brightly when we give and receive collectively. Embrace the mutual relationship between giving and receiving care. Encourage family, friends, colleagues, and organizations to take time for building resilience through conversation and support. Discuss the joys and challenges together to increase a sustainability that benefits everyone involved. Together, we find and develop a healthy common ground.

We never have to carry the world's sorrows and needs alone. Just think how dim the light of caring would be if that was the case. Our unique, individual paths connect and move toward a common goal of making the world a better place.

May we shed light on the beauty of caring for others while holding up hope radiating from shared strength and kindness. Now that we have looked at the various pieces of a sustainable journey, we will examine how the pieces fit together. A closer look at resilience can inspire and provide direction for the continued journey. The quest to apply resilient and sustainable caring practices is ongoing, but each small step can lead to big changes. Keep on shining inside and out!

GUIDE TO THRIVE STRATEGIES

1. Participate in an ongoing group focused on building resilience and sustainability.

2. Be intentional about choosing a sustainable work environment.

3. Foster supportive mentor and colleague relationships.

4. Process difficult events with others.

5. Find healing with a group of people facing similar struggles.

6. Expand your understanding of community to increase your support network.

Discussion Questions

What group processes do you think are helpful?

How do you define community?

What makes a community safe and supportive?

How can you increase a sense of community in your life?

What are the benefits of expanding community? What are the challenges?

Would you like to discuss any other ideas from the chapter?

Chapter 10

THRIVE WITH GROWING STRENGTH AND RESILIENCE

We can thrive with joy even amid the difficult.

See the Resilient and Sustainable Journey

I had a "Yes! That's resilient and sustainable caring!" moment a few months after leaving a difficult position that had taken a toll on my well-being. I had worked hard to promote sustainable caring, but the organization was too caught up in dysfunction, so I couldn't create the changes I needed to stay. My "Yes!" moment occurred while I was in Honduras working with a variety of projects, including a medical brigade. I felt as though I was walking in the sunshine on a clear path.

Resilient and sustainable caring doesn't mean the journey is without challenges or storms, but that we find more fulfillment than stress. We bounce back from difficulties with hope and purpose. We can go home after a long day and still have energy to play with the kids, take the dog on a walk, or cook a nice dinner. A coworker's stress or a patient's rudeness doesn't dominate how we see the day. We can support a family member without their struggle becoming our struggle.

Caring sustainably means we can be honest when we struggle with a difficult loss. Asking for help after making a mistake doesn't feel too frightening. We give ourselves a hug and say kind words when struggling, rather than berating ourselves. We share our opinion even when it is different from others, and we allow them to do the same. Resilient and sustainable caring means a lot of things, and it includes being authentic about what we believe and who we are. Our purpose provides more fuel than coffee or anxiety, so we face each day with renewed energy.

My recent moment of resilient and sustainable caring occurred after an intense day with a medical brigade. A line of people wrapped around the makeshift clinic in a Honduran mountain village. Women with young children holding on to their brightly colored skirts, elderly men with sombreros shading their eyes, and young adults wearing donated T-shirts from US events waited patiently for hours. Families had traveled by foot for miles to get the only medical help available.

Medical care providers and other helpers from the United States and Honduras turned a small school into a medical clinic for the day. Dentists set up lawn chairs for exams and tooth extractions. Physicians met with people in clusters of chairs and school desks in crowded rooms.

Among the busyness, a physician asked me to provide pastoral care to Juanita, a woman struggling with an abusive relationship. I followed him to his station, where she sat with her head bowed and hands in her lap. Juanita tearfully talked about how her husband hit her and called her names. He refused to let her go to church and other social gatherings, because he said, "God doesn't love you, so you don't deserve to go." She explained, "The last time he beat me so bad I thought for sure I was going to die. He will kill me."

We may be able to clearly see such abuse is not acceptable, but Juanita wasn't sure she deserved a better life. After all, that is what her husband screamed at her, and other people's complacency reinforced it. I tried to convince her she was worth caring about and should be treated differently, with kindness and respect.

While Juanita and I were talking, Larry, one of the brigade leaders, anxiously came into the room and yelled, "What are you doing here? Can't you see the long line of people waiting to see the doctor?" I had been focused on trying to help Juanita and was surprised by his anger.

We left the room and found the only space available—an area filled with children. As we continued our discussion, a small boy stood next to Juanita, and she sadly explained he was a kindred spirit. "His parents hit him, and I try to help him, because I know how hard it is."

Juanita sensed abuse was wrong, but she needed someone to affirm her suspicions and help her see a better way to live. I held her when she broke down in tears and prayed with her to reassure her of God's love. I don't know what she did after we talked, but I was hopeful our conversation gave her the courage to seek safety.

My time with Juanita was filled with emotions and meaning. I was exhausted and saddened by the abuse she, the boy, and others endure. I was disheartened to see such a lack of resources for so many people. I really wanted to change the world for them, but I felt helpless. I recalled Larry's outburst, and shame crept into the mix. The day's events reminded me of the challenges and pain I endured over the years. I had worked hard to bounce back from the toxic position I recently left, but it invaded the day's emotional mix.

I mindfully recognized how I was feeling, gave myself a hug, and said, "Later. I can deal with this later." After helping about four hundred people, we packed up the remaining supplies, put chairs away, and climbed into the buses ready to take us down the mountain.

I watched the mountain scenery change to fields of sugarcane and thought about the day. Amid the chaos of feelings, I remembered my purpose statement: *"I will glorify God and promote healthy living characterized by love, kindness, peace, honesty, and hope."* I prayed and meditated with a focus on compassion for myself. I replaced the negative internal dialogue running through my mind with positive, healing messages. I thought about healthy boundaries and what I was responsible for.

I cried healing tears and debated whether or not to confront Larry. Because we had worked together for such a short time, I decided not to and was able to let go of my anger and hurt. Talking with a friend outside of the group helped me process what happened and let go of the shame. I allowed myself to feel the mixture of brokenness from a hard day—hard year, really—but I also knew hope was present, even if I couldn't feel it at the moment. The following day, I felt as though a heavy weight was lifted off my shoulders, and I looked forward to new opportunities.

The day's challenges were just a bump in my journey. I was able to let go of what drained my energy and move forward to help others while promoting my best, balanced self. Moments of laughter and hugs overshadowed the heartache I experienced while being with people who endured abuse, families trying to survive poverty, and children struggling because of their parents' addictions. Moments of self-care supplemented meaningful connections to provide a bounce in my step.

I have discovered sustainable caring and am stronger than ever. Resilience is a faithful friend, and purpose has become my guiding light. I can help others while being grounded in what's important to reflect my best, balanced self. Self-compassion is now integral to daily life. I worked hard to forgive myself and others, and this has unchained me from past pain.

Anxiety inspires me to address challenges but does not rule my days. Conflict and loss will have a presence in life, but I believe I can face them with integrity and hope. Now, I can ask for help from an array of resources and a supportive community, and in doing so, I can experience the care we helpers try to shape the world with. My journey has been a long walk, but in many ways it's just beginning.

Use Guide to Thrive Strategies

Growing resilience and sustainability are part of a lifelong journey. Efforts to strengthen our best, balanced self, decrease anxiety, and expand support require ongoing attention but also can provide immediate relief. Strategies to thrive while caring include:

Strengthen Your Best, Balanced Self

- Develop awareness of support and shared challenges across helping roles globally.
- Articulate personal values, virtues, and purpose.
- Define what your best, balanced self looks like based on important values, virtues, and purpose, and help yourself demonstrate this in daily interactions.
- Establish and honor healthy boundaries.
- Foster compassion for self and others.
- Offer self-forgiveness to recover and learn from mistakes.

Decrease Anxiety and Increase the Ability to Regulate Emotions

- Increase self-differentiation to regulate anxiety.
- Decrease group anxiety.
- Choose life perspectives.
- Recognize and defuse emotional triggers.
- Be mindful and nourish spirituality to expand inner peace.
- Alter perception of conflict to increase constructive possibilities.
- Perceive and disrupt conflict patterns in groups.
- Change unhelpful conflict habits by using an array of skills.
- Build awareness of grief responses and ways to promote healthy recovery.

Expand Support

- Increase and use available resources.
- Develop opportunities to connect with others.
- Talk about challenges and vulnerabilities with safe people.
- Expand a sense of community.
- Be a safe person for others.
- Influence individuals and groups to be more resilient and sustainable.

Look at the Journey Ahead

Now that you have learned a variety of ways to increase resilience, you can create a more sustainable journey. I hope you find ongoing support and guidance from *Resilient and Sustainable Caring*. Making important life changes take time and determination. Everyone experiences challenges in trying to change. When life gets hard, we often slip into old habits, even though they may not be helpful. Take heart and remember even small changes make a big difference.

I hope to help you especially when change is hard to find or sustainability seems like a distant dream. Continue developing your own guide to thrive by adding pieces from *Resilient and Sustainable Caring* to your journey over time. Strategies that sing loudest to you will become second nature with practice. You can connect with concepts and tools for specific situations by revisiting applicable chapters. Be intentional about building balance and resilience.

Look for additional *Resilient and Sustainable Caring* resources, such as accompanying workbooks and daily reflections. Check out my website (karenschuder.com) for information on additional services, speaking engagements, or workshops. Let's make caring for others a more sustainable, joy-filled journey.

You transform the world with goodness while helping others. I am thankful for all you do to make the world a better place. You are a blessing and deserve the same care you offer to others. As you strengthen your best, balanced self, decrease anxiety, and expand support, you will find more joy and energy for the journey of helping others. Resilience and sustainability are a reality, not just a hope.

Resilience at Work: Imagine Your Sustainable Journey

Smiles and kindness nourish you on the journey of helping others. Tender moments create a respite, a pause to embrace meaning. Hardships and frustrations challenge progress sometimes, especially when accompanied by doubt and discouragement. You know the pull of resistance. Yet even at such times, a sense of purpose kicks in, and you continue the journey with determination. Not in a tired way, but with hopeful steps. When you are occasionally knocked down and it is hard to get back up, you reach out to find caring hearts offering a lift.

Through it all—you are grounded in purpose and peace. You know you can handle the difficult and still thrive.

Appendix A

Suggested Reading List

Chapter 2

Buckingham, Marcus, and Donald O. Clifton, PhD. *Now, Discover Your Strengths*. New York: Gallup Press, 2020.

Covey, Stephen R. *The 7 Habits of Highly Effective People: Powerful Lessons in Personal Change*. New York: Simon & Schuster, 1989.

Frankl, Viktor E. *Man's Search for Meaning: An Introduction to Logotherapy*. 3rd ed. New York: Simon & Schuster, 1984.

Gilbert, Roberta M. *Extraordinary Relationships: A New Way of Thinking about Human Interactions*. New York: John Wiley & Sons, Inc., 1992.

Senge, Peter M. *The Fifth Discipline: The Art and Practice of the Learning Organization*. New York: Doubleday, 2006.

Chapter 3

Cloud, Henry, and John Townsend. *Boundaries: When to Say Yes, How to Say No to Take Control of Your Life*. Grand Rapids, MI: Zondervan, 2017.

Gilbert, Roberta M. *The Eight Concepts of Bowen Theory*. Lake Frederick, VA: Leading Systems Press, 2004.

Manning, Shari Y. *Loving Someone with Borderline Personality Disorder: How to Keep Out-of-Control Emotions from Destroying Your Relationship*. New York: The Guilford Press, 2011.

Skovholt, Thomas M., and Michelle Trotter-Mathison. *The Resilient Practitioner: Burnout and Compassion Fatigue Prevention and Self-Care Strategies for the Helping Professions*. 3rd ed. New York: Routledge Taylor & Francis Group, 2016.

Chapter 4

Chodron, Pema. *Start Where You Are: A Guide to Compassionate Living*. Boulder, CO: Shambhala Publications, Inc., 1994.

Jinpa, Thupten. *A Fearless Heart: How the Courage to Be Compassionate Can Transform Our Lives*. New York: Avery, 2015.

Neff, Kristin. *Self-Compassion: The Proven Power of Being Kind to Yourself*. New York: Harper Collins Publishers, 2011.

Smedes, Lewis B. *The Art of Forgiving: When You Need to Forgive and Don't Know How*. New York: Ballantine Books, 1996.

Chapter 5

Brown, Jenny. *Growing Yourself Up: How to Bring Your Best to All of Life's Relationships*. 2nd ed. Dunedin, New Zealand: Exisle Publishing, 2017.

Dalai Lama, Desmond Tutu, and Douglas Abrams. *The Book of Joy: Lasting Happiness in a Changing World.* New York: Avery an imprint of Penguin Random House, 2016.

Hansel, Tim. *You Gotta Keep Dancin': In the Midst of Life's Hurts, You Can Choose Joy.* Elgin, IL: David C. Cook Publishing Co., 1985.

Kabat-Zinn, Jon. *Coming to Our Senses: Healing Ourselves and the World through Mindfulness.* New York: Hyperion, 2005.

Siegel, Daniel J. "Mindfulness Training and Neural Integration: Differentiation of Distinct Streams of Awareness and the Cultivation of Well-Being." *Social Cognitive and Affective Neuroscience* 2, no. 4 (December 2007): 259-263. https://doi.org/10.1093/scan/nsm034.

Chapter 6

Chaleff, Ira. *Intelligent Disobedience: Doing Right When What You're Told to Do Is Wrong.* Oakland, CA: Berrett-Koehler Publishers, Inc., 2015.

Lederach, John P. *The Little Book of Conflict Transformation: Clear Articulation of Guiding Principles by a Pioneer in the Field.* New York: Good Books, 2003.

Pachter, Barbara, and Susan Magee. *The Power of Positive Confrontation: The Skills You Need to Know to Handle Conflicts at Work, at Home, and in Life.* New York: Marlowe & Company, 2000.

Schrock-Schenk, Carolyn, and Lawrence Ressler, eds. *Making Peace with Conflict: Practical Skills for Conflict Transformation.* Harrisonburg, VA: Herald Press, 1999.

Tutu, Desmond, and Mpho Tutu. *The Book of Forgiving: The Fourfold Path for Healing Ourselves and Our World*. New York: Harper One, 2015.

Chapter 7

Bonanno, George A. *The Other Side of Sadness: What the New Science of Bereavement Tells Us about Life After Loss*. New York: Basic Books, 2009.

Kubler-Ross, Elizabeth, and David Kessler. *On Grief and Grieving: Finding the Meaning of Grief through the Five Stages of Loss*. New York: Simon & Schuster, 2005.

Noel, Brook, and Pamela D. Blair. *I Wasn't Ready to Say Goodbye: Surviving, Coping, and Healing After the Sudden Death of a Loved One*. Naperville, IL: Sourcebooks, Inc., 2018.

Westberg, Granger E. *Good Grief.* Philadelphia: Fortress Press, 1971.

Chapter 8

Brown, Brené. *The Gifts of Imperfection: Let Go of Who You Think You're Supposed to Be and Embrace Who You Are*. Center City, MN: Hazelden Publishing, 2010.

Graham, Linda. *Resilience: Powerful Practices for Bouncing Back from Disappointment, Difficulty, and Even Disaster*. Novato, CA: New World Library, 2018.

Van Dernoot Lipsky, Laura, and Connie Burk. *Trauma Stewardship: An Everyday Guide to Caring for Self While Caring for Others.* Oakland, CA: Berrett-Koehler Publishers, Inc., 2009.

Chapter 9

Hanson, Rick. *Resilient: How to Grow an Unshakable Core of Calm, Strength, and Happiness.* New York: Harmony Books, 2018.

Mitchell, Jeffrey T. "Critical Incident Stress Debriefing (CISD)." https://www.info-trauma.org/critical incident stress debriefing.

Palmer, Parker J. *A Hidden Wholeness: The Journey toward an Undivided Life.* San Francisco, CA: Jossey-Bass, 2004.

ENDNOTES

Chapter 1

1. Suzanne E. Tomasi, Ethan D. Fechter-Leggett, and Nicole T. Edwards, "Suicide Among Veterinarians in the United States from 1979 through 2015," *Journal of the American Veterinary Medical Association* 254, no. 1 (January 2019): 104-112. https://doi.org/10.2460/javma.254.1.104.

2. Sara Berg, "Physician Burnout: It's Not You, It's Your Medical Specialty," *American Medical Association*, accessed July 28, 2020, http://ama-assn.org.

3. Thomas P. Reith, "Burnout in United States Healthcare Professionals: A Narrative Review," *Cureus* 10, no.12 (December 4, 2018): e.3681, https://doi.org/10.7759/cureus.3681.

4. McCormack, Hannah M., Tadhg E. Macintyre, Deidre O'Shea, Matthew P. Herring, and Mark J. Campbell, "The Prevalence and Cause(s) of Burnout Among Applied Psychologists: A Systematic Review," *Frontiers in Psychology* 9, no.1897 (October 16, 2018): https://www.ncbi.nlm.nih.gov/pmc/ articles/PMC6198075/.

Simionato, Gabrielle K. and Susan Simpson, "Personal Risk Factors Associated with Burnout Among Psychotherapists: A Sytematic Review of Literature," *Journal of Clinical Psychology*

74, no.9 (March 24, 2018):1431-1456, https://doi.org/10.1002/jclp.22615.

5. Suhus Kulkarni, Dagli Namrata, Prabu Duraiswamy, Harshit Desai, Himanshu Vyas, and Kusai Baroudi, "Stress and Professional Burnout Among Newly Graduated Dentists," *Journal of International Society of Preventive & Community Dentistry* 6, no.6 (2016): 535-541, http:/www.jispcd.org.

6. Erich Barber, Chad Newland, Amy Young and Monique Rose, "Survey Reveals Alarming Rates of EMS Provider Stress and Thoughts of Suicide," *Journal of Emergency Medical Services* 10, no.40 (September 28, 2015), http://www.jems.com.

7. Virginia Held, *The Ethics of Care: Personal, Political and Global* (New York: Oxford University Press, 2006), 17.

8. Ayala Malakh-Pines, Elliot Aronson and Ditsa Kafry, *Burnout: From Tedium to Personal Growth* (New York: Free Press, 1981).

9. J. Eric Gentry, Anna Baranowsky and Kathleen Dunning. "The Accelerated Recovery Program (ARP) for Compassion Fatigue," *Psychosocial Stress Series: Treating Compassion Fatigue* ed. Charles Figley (Brunner-Routledge, 2002), 123-137.

10. Paul Valent, "Survival Strategies: A Framework for Understanding Secondary Traumatic Stress and Coping in Helpers," in *Compassion Fatigue: Coping with Secondary Traumatic Stress in Those Who Treat the Traumatized*, ed. Charles R. Figley (New York: Brunner/Mazel, Inc., 1995), 21-50.

11. Charles R. Figley, "Compassion Fatigue as Secondary Traumatic Stress Disorder: An Overview," in *Compassion Fatigue: Coping*

with Secondary Traumatic Stress in Those Who Treat the Traumatized, ed. Charles R. Figley (New York: Brunner/Mazel, Inc., 1995), 1-20.

12. Charles R. Figley, "Compassion Fatigue as Secondary Traumatic Stress Disorder."

13. Francois Mathieu, *The Compassion Fatigue Workbook: Creative Tools for Transforming Compassion Fatigue and Vicarious Traumatization* (New York: Routledge, 2012).

14. Charles R. Figley, "Compassion Fatigue as Secondary Traumatic Stress Disorder."

15. Mathieu, *The Compassion Fatigue Workbook.*

    Haleigh H. Barnes, Robin A. Hurley, and Katherine H. Taber, "Moral Injury and PTSD: Often Co-Occurring Yet Mechanistically Different," *Journal of Neuropsychiatry and Clinical Neurosciences* 31, no.2 (Spring 2019): 98-103, https://doi.org/10.1176/appi. neuropsych. 19020036.

16. Kimyon, Rebecca S., "Imposter Syndrome," *American Medical Association Journal of Ethics* 22, no.7, accessed July 27,2020, http://www.journalofethics.org.

    Weir, Kirsten, "Feel Like a Fraud? You're Not Alone. Many Graduate Students Question Whether They Are Prepared to Do the Work They Do. Here's How to Overcome that Feeling and Recognize Your Strengths," *American Psychological Association*, accessed July 27, 2020, http://www.apa.org.

17. Emee Vida Estacio, *The Imposter Syndrome Remedy: How to Improve Your Self-Worth, Feel Confident About Yourself, and Stop Feeling Like a Fraud* (www.thepamecode.com, 2018).

18. "Friedrich Nietzsche Quotes," *Brainy Quote*, accessed July 29, 2020, https://www.brainyquote.com/authors/friedrich-nietzsche-quotes. Used inclusive language.

19. Parker Palmer, *Let Your Life Speak: Listening for the Voice of Vocation* (San Francisco, CA: Jossey-Bass, 1999), 30.

Chapter 2

1. Michael E. Kerr & Murray Bowen, *Family Evaluation: The Role of the Family as an Emotional Unit that Governs Individual Behavior and Development* (New York: W.W. Norton & Company, 1988).

2. Roberta M. Gilbert, *The Eight Concepts of Bowen Theory* (Lake Frederick, VA: Leading Systems Press, 2004).

3. Jenny Brown, *Growing Yourself Up: How to Bring Your Best to All of Life's Relationships,* 2nd ed. (Dunedin, New Zealand: Exisle Publishing, 2017).

4. Edwin H. Friedman, *Reinventing Leadership: Discussion Guide* (New York: The Guilford Press, 1996).

5. Gilbert, *Eight Concepts.*

6. Roberta M. Gilbert, *Extraordinary Relationships: A New Way of Thinking about Human Interactions* (New York: John Wiley & Sons, Inc., 1992).

7. Edwin H. Friedman, *Generation to Generation: Family Process in Church and Synagogue* (New York, NY: The Guilford Press, 1985).

8. Karen L. Schuder, "Qualitative Study of Business Ethics Education: Preparing Leaders to Make Ethical Decisions," (EdD diss., University of St. Thomas, 2014).

9. Roberto Assagioli, *Cheerfulness (A Psychosynthesis Technique)* written 1973, accessed June 26, 2020, https://kennethsorensen.dk/en/.

10. Rachel N. Remen, *Kitchen Table Wisdom: Stories That Heal* (New York: Penguin Group Inc., 2006), 162.

11. Thomas M. Skovholt, and Michelle Trotter-Mathison, *The Resilient Practitioner: Burnout and Compassion Fatigue Prevention and Self-Care Strategies for the Helping Professions,* 3rd ed. (New York: Routledge, 2016).

12. Peter M. Senge, *The Fifth Discipline: The Art and Practice of the Learning Organization* (New York: Doubleday, 2006).

13. Stacey M. Schaefer, Jennifer Morozink Boylan, Carien M. van Reekum, Regina C. Lapate, Catherine J. Norris, Carol D. Ryff, and Richard J. Davidson, "Purpose in Life Predicts Better Emotional Recovery from Negative Stimuli," *PLOS ONE* 8, no.11 (November 2014), https://doi.org/10.1371/journal.pone.0080329

14. Viktor E. Frankl, *Man's Search for Meaning: An Introduction to Logotherapy,* 3rd ed. (New York: Simon & Schuster, 1984), 84.

15. Gordon Marino, *Ethics: The Essential Writings* (New York: Modern Library, 2010).

16. Justin Humphreys, "Artistotle: Ethics," *Internet Encyclopedia of Philosophy,* accessed June 29, 2020, https://iep.utm.edu/aristotle/.

17. Albert L. Winseman, Donald O. Clifton, and Curt Liesveld, *Living Your Strengths* (Washington D.C.: The Gallup Organization, 2003).

18. Winseman, Clifton, and Liesveld, *Living Your Strengths.*

19. Kerr and Bowen, *Family Evaluation.*

20. Stephen R. Covey, *The 7 Habits of Highly Effective People: Powerful Lessons in Personal Change* (New York: Simon & Schuster, 1989).

21. Laura van Dernoot Lipsky and Connie Burk, *Trauma Stewardship: An Everyday Guide to Caring for Self While Caring for Others* (Oakland, CA: Berrett-Koehler Publishers, Inc., 2009).

22. Senge, *The Fifth Discipline.*

23. Schuder, "Qualitative Study of Business Ethics Education."

24. Schuder, "Qualitative Study of Business Ethics Education."

25. Van Dernoot Lipsky and Burk, *Trauma Stewardship.*

Chapter 3

1. Michael E. Kerr & Murray Bowen, *Family Evaluation: The Role of the Family as an Emotional Unit that Governs Individual Behavior and Development* (New York: W.W. Norton & Company, 1988).

2. Linda Graham, *Resilience: Powerful Practices for Bouncing Back from Disappointment, Difficulty, and Even Disaster* (Novato, CA: New World Library, 2018).

3. Jenny Brown, *Growing Yourself Up: How to Bring Your Best to All of Life's Relationships,* 2nd ed. (Dunedin, New Zealand: Exisle Publishing, 2017).

4. Edwin H. Friedman, *Generation to Generation: Family Process in Church and Synagogue* (New York, NY: The Guilford Press, 1985).

5. Henry Cloud and John Townsend, *Boundaries: When to Say Yes, How to Say No to Take Control of Your Life* (Grand Rapids, MI: Zondervan, 2017).

6. Janet Yassen, "Preventing Secondary Traumatic Stress Disorder" in *Compassion Fatigue: Coping with Secondary Traumatic Stress in Those Who Treat the Traumatized,* ed. Charles R. Figley (New York: Brunner/Mazel, Inc., 1995), 178-208.

7. Friedman, *Generation to Generation.*

8. Cloud and Townsend, *Boundaries.*

9. Karen L. Schuder, "Qualitative Study of Business Ethics Education: Preparing Leaders to Make Ethical Decisions," (EdD diss., University of St. Thomas, 2014).

10. Thomas M. Skovholt, and Michelle Trotter-Mathison, *The Resilient Practitioner: Burnout and Compassion Fatigue Prevention and Self-Care Strategies for the Helping Professions,* 3rd ed. (New York: Routledge, 2016).

11. Kerr and Bowen, *Family Evaluation.*

12. "Empathy," *Online Etymology Dictionary,* accessed October 13, 2021, https://www.etymonline.com.

13. Skovholt and Trotter-Mathison, *The Resilient Practitioner.*

14. Brené Brown, *I Thought It Was Just Me (But It Isn't): Making the Journey from "What Will People Think?" to "I am Enough"* (New York: Gotham, 2007).

   Rick Hanson, *Resilient: How to Grow an Unshakable Core of Calm, Strength, and Happiness* (New York: Harmony, 2018).

15. Kerr and Bowen, *Family Evaluation.*

16. Thupten Jinpa, *A Fearless Heart: How the Courage to Be Compassionate Can Transform Our Lives* (New York: Avery, 2015).

17. Friedman, *Generation to Generation.*

18. Jinpa, *A Fearless Heart.*

19. Roberta M. Gilbert, *Extraordinary Relationships: A New Way of Thinking about Human Interactions* (New York: John Wiley & Sons, Inc., 1992).

20. Kerr and Bowen, *Family Evaluation.*

21. Jenny Brown, *Growing Yourself Up: How to Bring Your Best to All of Life's Relationships,* 2nd ed. (Dunedin, New Zealand: Exisle Publishing, 2017).

22. Laura van Dernoot Lipsky and Connie Burk, *Trauma Stewardship: An Everyday Guide to Caring for Self While Caring for Others* (Oakland, CA: Berrett-Koehler Publishers, Inc., 2009).

23. Gilbert, *Extraordinary Relationships.*

24. Hanson, *Resilient;* Skovholt and Trotter-Mathison, *The Resilient Practitioner.*

25. Cloud and Townsend, *Boundaries.*

26. Cloud and Townsend, *Boundaries.*

27. Shari Y. Manning, *Loving Someone with Borderline Personality Disorder: How to Keep Out-of-Control Emotions from Destroying Your Relationship* (New York: The Guilford Press, 2011).

28. Manning, *Loving Someone with Borderline Personality Disorder.*

29. Kerr and Bowen, *Family Evaluation.*

30. Manning, *Loving Someone with Borderline Personality Disorder.*

31. Cloud and Townsend, *Boundaries.*

32. Manning, *Loving Someone with Borderline Personality Disorder.*

33. Cloud and Townsend, *Boundaries.*

34. Manning, *Loving Someone with Borderline Personality Disorder.*

35. Madeleine L'Engle, *A Circle of Quiet: The Crosswicks Journal.* (New York: Farrar, Straus and Giroux, 1972), 22.

Chapter 4

1. Kristin Neff, *Self-Compassion: The Proven Power of Being Kind to Yourself* (New York: Harper Collins Publishers, 2011).

2. Pema Chodron, *Start Where You Are: A Guide to Compassionate Living* (Boulder, CO: Shambhala Publications, Inc., 1994).

3. Dalai Lama, Desmond. Tutu, and Douglas Abrams, *The Book of Joy: Lasting Happiness in a Changing World* (New York: Avery, 2016), 254.

4. Thupten Jinpa, *A Fearless Heart: How the Courage to Be Compassionate Can Transform Our Lives* (New York: Avery, 2015).

5. Norman Fischer, *Training in Compassion: Zen Teachings on the Practice of Lojong* (Boston, MA: Shambhala Publications, 2013).

6. Chodron, *Start Where You Are.*

7. Neff, *Self-Compassion.*

8. Jinpa, *A Fearless Heart.*

9. Neff, *Self-Compassion.*

10. Neff, *Self-Compassion.*

11. Christopher Germer and Kristin Neff, *Teaching the Mindful Self-Compassion Program: A Guide for Professionals* (New York: The Guilford Press, 2019).

12. Jinpa, *A Fearless Heart.*

13. Neff, *Self-Compassion.*

14. Neff, *Self-Compassion*; Jinpa, *A Fearless Heart.*

15. Neff, *Self-Compassion.*

16. Brene' Brown, *I Thought It Was Just Me (But It Isn't): Making the Journey from "What Will People Think?* (New York: Avery, 2007).

   Lewis B. Smedes, *Shame and Grace: Healing the Shame We Don't Deserve* (New York: Harper One, 1993).

17. Brene' Brown, *The Gifts of Imperfection: Let Go of Who You Think You're Supposed to Be and Embrace Who You Are* (Center City, MN: Hazelden Publishing, 2010).

18. Chodron, *Start Where You Are.*

19. Reinhold Niebuhr, "The Irony of American History," *Major Works on Religion and Politics* (New York: Library Classics of the United States,2015), 705.

20. Tara Brach, *Radical Compassion: Learning to Love Yourself and Your World with the Practice of RAIN* (New York: Viking Life, 2019).

21. Brown, *The Gifts of Imperfection.*

22. Germer and Neff, *Teaching the Mindful Self-Compassion Program.*

23. Jon Kabat-Zinn, *Coming to Our Senses: Healing Ourselves and the World Through Mindfulness* (New York: Hyperion, 2005).

24. Thomas M. Skovholt, and Michelle Trotter-Mathison, *The Resilient Practitioner: Burnout and Compassion Fatigue Prevention and Self-Care Strategies for the Helping Professions,* 3rd ed. (New York: Routledge, 2016).

25. Edwin H. Friedman, *Generation to Generation: Family Process in Church and Synagogue.* (New York, NY: The Guilford Press, 1985).

26. Kabat-Zinn, *Coming to Our Senses.*

27. Germer and Neff, *Teaching the Mindful Self-Compassion Program.*

28. Brown, *The Gifts of Imperfection.*

29. Neff, *Self-Compassion*.

30. Hanson, Rick, *Resilient: How to Grow an Unshakable Core of Calm, Strength, and Happiness* (New York: Harmony Books, 2018).

Neff, *Self-Compassion*.

31. Desmond TuTu and Mpho Tutu, *The Book of Forgiving: The Fourfold Path for Healing Ourselves and Our World* (New York: Harper One, 2014).

32. Neff, *Self-Compassion*.

33. Lewis B. Smedes, *The Art of Forgiving: When You Need to Forgive and Don't Know How* (New York: Ballantine Books, 1996).

34. Smedes, *The Art of Forgiving*.

35. Smedes, *The Art of Forgiving*.

36. Neff, *Self-Compassion*.

37. Neff, *Self-Compassion*.

Chapter 5

1. Robert M. Sapolsky, *Why Zebras Don't Get Ulcers: The Acclaimed Guide to Stress, Stress-Related Diseases, and Coping*, 3rd ed. (New York: St. Martin's Griffin, 1998).

2. Sapolsky, *Why Zebras Don't Get Ulcers*.

3. Mike Dubi, Patrick Powell, and J. Eric Gentry, *Trauma, PTSD, Grief & Loss: The 10 Core Competencies for Evidence-Based Treatment* (Eau Claire, WI: PESI Publishing & Media, 2017).

4. Sapolsky, *Why Zebras Don't Get Ulcers.*

5. Dubi, Powell, and Gentry, *Trauma PTSD, Grief and Loss.*

6. Sapolsky, *Why Zebras Don't Get Ulcers.*

7. Michael E. Kerr & Murray Bowen, *Family Evaluation: The Role of the Family as an Emotional Unit that Governs Individual Behavior and Development* (New York: W.W. Norton & Company, 1988).

8. Sapolsky, *Why Zebras Don't Get Ulcers.*

9. Kerr and Bowen, *Family Evaluation.*

10. Roberta M. Gilbert, *The Eight Concepts of Bowen Theory* (Lake Frederick, VA: Leading Systems Press, 2004).

11. Kerr and Bowen, *Family Evaluation.*

12. Jenny Brown, *Growing Yourself Up: How to Bring Your Best to All of Life's Relationships,* 2nd ed. (Dunedin, New Zealand: Exisle Publishing, 2017).

13. Roberta M. Gilbert, *Extraordinary Relationships: A New Way of Thinking about Human Interactions* (New York: John Wiley & Sons, Inc., 1992).

14. Gilbert, *The Eight Concepts of Bowen Theory.*

15. Gilbert, *Extraordinary Relationships.*

16. Edwin H. Friedman, *Generation to Generation: Family Process in Church and Synagogue* (New York, NY: The Guilford Press, 1985).

17. Roberta M. Gilbert, *Extraordinary Leadership: Thinking Systems, Making a Difference* (Falls Church, VA: Leading Systems Press, 2006).

18. Daniel J. Siegel, "Mindfulness Training and Neural Integration: Differentiation of Distinct Streams of Awareness and the Cultivation of Well-Being," *Social Cognitive and Affective Neuroscience (SCAN) 2, no.4* (2007): 259-263, https://doi.org/10.1093/scan/nsm034.

19. Jane Yolen, ed., "The Missing Axe," in *Favorite Folktales from Around the World* (New York: Pantheon Books, 1986), 412.

20. Linda Graham, *Resilience: Powerful Practices for Bouncing Back from Disappointment, Difficulty, and Even Disaster* (Novato, CA: New World Library, 2018).

21. Seligman, *Flourish.*

22. Tim Hansel, *You Gotta Keep Dancin': In the Midst of Life's Hurts, You Can Choose Joy* (Elgin, IL: David C. Cook Publishing Co., 1985), 55.

23. Dalai Lama, Desmond. Tutu, and Douglas Abrams, *The Book of Joy: Lasting Happiness in a Changing World* (New York: Avery, 2016), 11.

24. Jonathan Haidt, *The Happiness Hypothesis: Finding Modern Truth in Ancient Wisdom* (New York: Basic Books, 2006).

25. Mike Dubi, Patrick Powell, and J. Eric Gentry, *Trauma, PTSD, Grief & Loss: The 10 Core Competencies for Evidence-Based Treatment* (Eau Claire, WI: PESI Publishing & Media, 2017).

26. Lane Pederson and Cortney Sidwell Pederson, *The Expanded Dialectical Behavior Therapy Skills Training Manual: DBT for Self-Help, and Individual & Group Treatment Settings* (Eau Claire, WI: PESI Publishing & Media, 2017).

27. Jon Kabat-Zinn, *Coming to Our Senses: Healing Ourselves and the World Through Mindfulness* (New York: Hyperion, 2005).

28. Sapolsky, *Why Zebras Don't Get Ulcers.*

29. Edwin H. Friedman, *Reinventing Leadership: Discussion Guide* (New York: The Guilford Press, 1996).

30. Laura van Dernoot Lipsky and Connie Burk, *Trauma Stewardship: An Everyday Guide to Caring for Self While Caring for Others* (Oakland, CA: Berrett-Koehler Publishers, Inc., 2009).

31. Siegel, *Mindfulness Training and Neural Integration.*

32. Kabat-Zinn, *Coming to Our Senses.*

33. Kabat-Zinn, *Coming to Our Senses,* 7.

34. Pederson and Sidwell Pederson, *The Expanded Dialectical Behavior Therapy Skills Training Manual.*

35. Laurel Parnell, *Tapping In: A Step-by-Step Guide to Activating Your Healing Resources Through Bilateral Stimulation* (Boulder, Co: Sounds True, 2008).

36. Haidt, *The Happiness Hypothesis.*

37. Thomas M. Skovholt, and Michelle Trotter-Mathison, *The Resilient Practitioner: Burnout and Compassion Fatigue Prevention and Self-Care Strategies for the Helping Professions,* 3rd ed. (New York: Routledge, 2016).

38. Sapolsky, *Why Zebras Don't Get Ulcers*.

39. Friedman, *Generation to Generation*; Gilbert, *Extraordinary Leadership*.

40. Friedman, *Generation to Generation*; Gilbert, *Extraordinary Leadership*.

41. Kerr and Bowen, *Family Evaluation*.

42. Aviezer Ravitzky, "Shalom: Peace in Hebrew," *Contemporary Jewish Religious Thought*, accessed October 23, 2020, https://www.myjewishlearning.com/ article/shalom/.

Chapter 6

1. Robert M. Sapolsky, *Why Zebras Don't Get Ulcers: The Acclaimed Guide to Stress, Stress-Related Diseases, and Coping*, 3rd ed. (New York: St. Martin's Griffin, 1998).

2. Carolyn Schrock-Schenk, "Introducing Conflict and Conflict Transformation," in *Making Peace with Conflict: Practical Skills for Conflict Transformation*, eds. Carolyn Schrock-Schenk and Lawrence Ressler (Harrisonburg, VA: Herald Press, 1999), 25-37.

3. David W. Augsberger, *Conflict Mediation Across Cultures: Pathways and Patterns* (Louisville, KY: Westminster/John Knox Press, 1992).

4. Michael E. Kerr & Murray Bowen, *Family Evaluation: The Role of the Family as an Emotional Unit that Governs Individual Behavior and Development* (New York: W.W. Norton & Company, 1988).

5. Edwin H. Friedman, *Generation to Generation: Family Process in Church and Synagogue* (New York: The Guilford Press, 1985).

6. Schrock-Schenk, "Introducing Conflict and Conflict Transformation."

7. John Paul Lederach, *The Little Book of Conflict Transformation: Clear Articulation of Guiding Principles by a Pioneer in the Field* (New York: Good Books, 2003).

8. Sapolsky, *Why Zebras Don't Get Ulcers*.

9. Victor E. Frankl, *Man's Search for Meaning: An Introduction to Logotherapy*, 3rd ed. (New York: Simon & Schuster, 1984), 75.

10. Schrock-Shenk, "Introducing Conflict and Conflict Transformation."

11. Kerr and Bowen, *Family Evaluation*.

12. Roberta M. Gilbert, *The Eight Concepts of Bowen Theory* (Lake Frederick, VA: Leading Systems Press, 2004).

13. Friedman, *Generation to Generation*.

14. Kerr and Bowen, *Family Evaluation*.

15. Augsberger, *Conflict Mediation Across Cultures*.

16. Peter L. Steinke, *Congregational Leadership in Anxious Times: Being Calm and Courageous No Matter What* (Herndon, VA: The Alban Institute, 2006).

17. Kerr and Bowen, *Family Evaluation*.

18. Augsberger, *Conflict Mediation Across Cultures*.

19. Lederach, *Little Book of Conflict Transformation*.

20. Alan E. Fruzzetti, *The High-Conflict Couple: A Dialectical Behavior Therapy Guide to Finding Peace, Intimacy and Validation* (Oakland, CA: New Harbinger Publications, Inc., 2006).

21. John Paul Lederach, *Reconcile: Conflict Transformation for Ordinary Christians* (Harrisonburg, VA: Herald Press, 2014).

22. Augsberger, *Conflict Mediation Across Cultures*.

23. Kori Leaman-Miller, "Listening," in *Making Peace with Conflict: Practical Skills for Conflict Transformation*, eds. Carolyn Schrock-Schenk and Lawrence Ressler (Harrisonburg, VA: Herald Press, 1999), 59-67.

24. Barbara Pachter and Susan Magee, *The Power of Positive Confrontation: The Skills You Need to Know to Handle Conflicts at Work, at Home, and in Life* (New York: Marlowe & Company, 2000).

25. Valerie Weaver-Zercher, "Speaking," in *Making Peace with Conflict: Practical Skills for Conflict Transformation*, eds. Carolyn Schrock-Schenk and Lawrence Ressler (Harrisonburg, VA: Herald Press, 1999), 68-76.

26. Pachter and Magee, *The Power of Positive Confrontation*.

27. Augsberger, *Conflict Mediation Across Cultures*.

28. Pachter and Magee, *The Power of Positive Confrontation*.

29. Augsberger, *Conflict Mediation Across Cultures*.

30. Augsberger, *Conflict Mediation Across Cultures*.

31. Fruzzetti, *The High-Conflict Couple*.

32. Shari Y. Manning, *Loving Someone with Borderline Personality Disorder: How to Keep Out-of-Control Emotions from Destroying Your Relationship* (New York: The Guilford Press, 2011).

33. Kerr and Bowen, *Family Evaluation.*

34. Manning, *Loving Someone with Borderline Personality.*

35. Manning, *Loving Someone with Borderline Personality.*

36. Ira Chaleff, *The Courageous Follower: Standing Up To and For Our Leaders*, 3rd ed. (San Francisco: Berrett-Koehler Publishers, Inc.,2009).

37. Ira Chaleff, *Intelligent Disobedience: Doing Right When What You're Told to Do Is Wrong* (Oakland, CA: Berrett-Koehler Publishers, Inc., 2015), 2.

38. Roberta M. Gilbert, *Extraordinary Leadership: Thinking Systems, Making a Difference* (Falls Church, VA: Leading Systems Press, 2006).

39. Gilbert, *Extraordinary Leadership.*

40. Augsberger, *Conflict Mediation Across Cultures.*

41. Lederach, *Reconcile.*

42. Corrie ten Boom, John Sherrill, and Elizabeth Sherrill, *The Hiding Place* (Old Tappan, New Jersey: Fleming H. Revell Company Spire Books. 1971), 238.

43. Lederach, *Reconcile.*

44. Augsberger, *Conflict Mediation Across Cultures.*

45. Desmond TuTu and Mpho Tutu, *The Book of Forgiving: The Fourfold Path for Healing Ourselves and Our World* (New York: Harper One, 2014), 25.

Chapter 7

1. Geert Hofstede, Gert Jan Hofstede, and Michael Minkov, *Cultures and organizations: Software of the mind*, 3rd ed. (New York, NY: McGraw-Hill, 2010).

2. Edgar H. Schein, *Organizational Culture and Leadership*, 3rd ed. (San Francisco, CA: Jossey Bass, 2004).

3. George A. Bonanno, *The Other Side of Sadness: What the New Science of Bereavement Tells Us About Life After Loss* (New York: Basic Books, 2009).

4. Elizabeth Kubler-Ross and David Kessler, *On Grief and Grieving: Finding the Meaning of Grief Through the Five Stages of Loss* (New York: Simon & Schuster, 2005).

5. Mike Dubi, Patrick Powell, and J. Eric Gentry, *Trauma, PTSD, Grief & Loss: The 10 Core Competencies for Evidence-Based Treatment* (Eau Claire, WI: PESI Publishing & Media, 2017).

6. J. William Worden, *Grief Counseling and Grief Therapy: A Handbook for the Mental Health Practitioner*, 4th ed. (New York: Springer Publishing Company, 2008).

7. Bonanno, *The Other Side of Sadness*.

8. Bonanno, *The Other Side of Sadness*.

9. C.S. Lewis, *A Grief Observed* (New York: Harper Collins, 1996), 60.

10. Kubler-Ross and Kessler, *On Grief and Grieving*.

11. Brook Noel and Pamela D. Blair, *I Wasn't Ready to Say Goodbye: Surviving, Coping, and Healing After the Sudden Death of a Loved One* (Naperville, IL: Sourcebooks, Inc., 2018).

12. Bonanno, *The Other Side of Sadness*; Kubler-Ross and Kessler, *On Grief and Grieving*.

13. Kubler-Ross and Kessler, *On Grief and Grieving*.

14. Noel and Blair, *I Wasn't Ready to Say Goodbye*.

15. Kubler-Ross and Kessler, *On Grief and Grieving*.

16. Kubler-Ross and Kessler, *On Grief and Grieving*.

17. Kubler-Ross and Kessler, *On Grief and Grieving*.

18. Kubler-Ross and Kessler, *On Grief and Grieving*.

19. Noel and Blair, *I Wasn't Ready to Say Goodbye*.

20. Kubler-Ross and Kessler, *On Grief and Grieving*.

21. Bonanno, *The Other Side of Sadness*.

22. H. Norman Wright, *Recovering from Losses in Life* (Grand Rapids, MI: Fleming H. Revell, 2006).

23. Wright, *Recovering from Losses in Life*.

24. Bonanno, *The Other Side of Sadness*.

25. Wright, *Recovering from Losses in Life*.

26. Bonanno, *The Other Side of Sadness.*

27. Linda Graham, *Resilience: Powerful Practices for Bouncing Back from Disappointment, Difficulty, and Even Disaster* (Novato, CA: New World Library, 2018).

28. Noel and Blair, *I Wasn't Ready to Say Goodbye.*

29. Noel and Blair, *I Wasn't Ready to Say Goodbye.*

30. Noel and Blair, *I Wasn't Ready to Say Goodbye.*

31. Roberta M. Gilbert, *Extraordinary Relationships: A New Way of Thinking about Human Interactions* (New York: John Wiley & Sons, Inc., 1992).

    Michael E. Kerr & Murray Bowen, *Family Evaluation: The Role of the Family as an Emotional Unit that Governs Individual Behavior and Development* (New York: W.W. Norton & Company, 1988).

32. Gilbert, *Extraordinary Relationships*; Kerr and Bowen, *Family Evaluation.*

33. Wright, *Recovering from Losses in Life.*

34. Noel and Blair, *I Wasn't Ready to Say Goodbye.*

35. Granger E. Westberg, *Good Grief* (Philadelphia: Fortress Press, 1971).

36. Noel and Blair, *I Wasn't Ready to Say Goodbye.*

37. Kubler-Ross and Kessler, *On Grief and Grieving.*

38. Rick Hanson, *Resilient: How to Grow an Unshakable Core of Calm, Strength, and Happiness* (New York: Harmony Books, 2018).

Chapter 8

1. "How Big are Big Trees?" California Department of Parks and Recreation, accessed March 7, 2022, https://www.parks.ca.gov/.

2. Don R. Catherall, "Coping with Secondary Traumatic Stress: The Importance of the Therapist's Professional Peer Group" in *Secondary Traumatic Stress: Self-Care Issues for Clinicians, Researchers, and Educators,* 2nd ed., ed. B. Hudnall Stamm (Baltimore, MD: Sidran Press, 1999), 80-92.

3. Janet Yassen, "Preventing Secondary Traumatic Stress Disorder" in *Compassion Fatigue: Coping with Secondary Traumatic Stress in Those Who Treat the Traumatized,* ed. Charles R. Figley (New York: Brunner/Mazel, Inc., 1995), 178-208.

4. Fabrizio Bert, Maria Rosaria Gualano, Elisa Camussi, Giulio Pieve, Gianluca Voglino, and Roberta Siliquini "Animal Assisted Intervention: A Systematic Review of Benefits and Risks," *European Journal of Integrative Medicine* 8, no.5 (May 2016): 695-706, http://dx.doi.org/10.1016/j.eujim.2016.05.005.

5. Dessa Bergen-Cico, Yvonne Smith, Karen Wolford, Collin Gooley, Kathleen Hannon, Ryan Woodruff, Melissa Spicer, and Brooks Gump, "Dog Ownership and Training Reduces Post-Traumatic Stress Symptoms and Increases Self-Compassion Among Veterans: Results of a Longitudinal Control Study," *J Altern Complement Med* 24, no.12 (December 2018): 1166-1175, https://pubmed.ncbi.nlm.nih.gov/30256652/.

6. Laura van Dernoot Lipsky, and Connie Burk, *Trauma Stewardship: An Everyday Guide to Caring for Self While Caring for Others* (Oakland, CA: Berrett-Koehler Publishers, Inc., 2009).

7. Thomas M. Skovholt, and Michelle Trotter-Mathison, *The Resilient Practitioner: Burnout and Compassion Fatigue Prevention and Self-Care Strategies for the Helping Professions,* 3rd ed. (New York: Routledge, 2016).

8. Brene' Brown, *The Gifts of Imperfection: Let Go of Who You Think You're Supposed to Be and Embrace Who You Are* (Center City, MN: Hazelden Publishing, 2010), 50.

9. Brown, *The Gifts of Imperfection.*

10. Michael E. Kerr and Murray Bowen, *Family Evaluation: The Role of Family as an Emotional Unit That Governs Individual Behaviors and Development* (New York: W.W. Norton & Company, 1988).

11. Parker Palmer, *A Hidden Wholeness: The Journey Toward an Undivided Life* (San Francisco, CA: Jossey-Bass, 2004), 5.

12. Skovholt and Trotter-Mathison, *The Resilient Practitioner.*

13. Kristin Neff, *Self-Compassion: The Proven Power of Being Kind to Yourself* (New York: Harper Collins Publishers, 2011).

14. Roberta M. Gilbert, *The Eight Concepts of Bowen Theory* (Lake Frederick, VA: Leading Systems Press, 2004).

15. Linda Graham, *Resilience: Powerful Practices for Bouncing Back from Disappointment, Difficulty, and Even Disaster* (Novato, CA: New World Library, 2018).

16. Yassen, *Preventing Secondary Traumatic Stress.*

17. Brown, *The Gifts of Imperfection.*

18. Brown, *The Gifts of Imperfection.*

19. Rachel Naomi Remen, *Kitchen Table Wisdom: Stories That Heal* (New York: Riverhead Books, 2006).

20. Brown, *The Gifts of Imperfection*.

21. Graham, *Resilience*.

22. Jenny Brown, *Growing Yourself Up: How to Bring Your Best to All of Life's Relationships*, 2nd ed. (Chatswood, Australia: Exisle Publishing, 2012).

23. Karen L. Schuder, "Qualitative Study of Business Ethics Education: Preparing Leaders to Make Ethical Decisions" (EdD diss., University of St. Thomas, 2014).

24. Francoise Mathieu, *The Compassion Fatigue Workbook: Creative Tools for Transforming Compassion Fatigue and Vicarious Traumatization* (New York: Routledge Taylor and Francis Group, 2012).

25. Sonya B. Norman and Shira Maguen, "Moral Injury," National Center for PTSD, accessed July 28, 2020, http://www.ptsd.va.gov.

26. Schuder, "Qualitative Study of Business Ethics Education."

27. Graham, *Resilience*.

28. Mathieu, *The Compassion Fatigue Workbook*.

29. Kerr and Bowen, *Family Evaluation*.

30. Skovholt and Trotter-Mathison, *The Resilient Practitioner*.

Chapter 9

1. "Split Rock Lighthouse," Minnesota Historical Society, accessed August 4, 2021, https://www.mnhs.org/splitrock.

2. Euan Kerr, "36 Years of Shining a Light on Split Rock's History Comes to an End," MPR News, last modified April 10, 2019, https://www.mprnews.org.

3. Janet Yassen, "Preventing Secondary Traumatic Stress Disorder" in *Compassion Fatigue: Coping with Secondary Traumatic Stress in Those Who Treat the Traumatized*, ed. Charles R. Figley (New York: Brunner/Mazel, Inc., 1995), 178-208.

4. Brene' Brown, *The Gifts of Imperfection: Let Go of Who You Think You're Supposed to Be and Embrace Who You Are* (Center City, MN: Hazelden Publishing, 2010).

5. Don R. Catherall, "Preventing Institutional Secondary Traumatic Stress Disorder," in *Compassion Fatigue: Coping with Secondary Traumatic Stress in Those Who Treat the Traumatized*, ed. Charles R. Figley (New York: Brunner/Mazel, Inc., 1995), 232-247.

6. Thomas M. Skovholt, and Michelle Trotter-Mathison, *The Resilient Practitioner: Burnout and Compassion Fatigue Prevention and Self-Care Strategies for the Helping Professions,* 3rd ed. (New York: Routledge, 2016).

7. Skovholt and Trotter-Mathison, *The Resilient Practitioner.*

8. James F. Munroe, Jonathan Shay, Lisa Fisher, Christine Makary, Kathryn Rapperport, and Rose Zimering, "Preventing Compassion Fatigue: A Team Treatment Model," in *Compassion Fatigue:*

Coping with Secondary Traumatic Stress in Those Who Treat the Traumatized, ed. Charles R. Figley (New York: Brunner/Mazel, Inc., 1995), 209-231.

9. Rick Hanson, *Resilient: How to Grow an Unshakable Core of Calm, Strength, and Happiness* (New York: Harmony Books, 2018).

10. Laura van Dernoot Lipsky, and Connie Burk, *Trauma Stewardship: An Everyday Guide to Caring for Self While Caring for Others* (Oakland, CA: Berrett-Koehler Publishers, Inc., 2009).

11. Randal D. Beaton, and Shirley A. Murphy, "Working with People in Crisis: Research Implications," in *Compassion Fatigue: Coping with Secondary Traumatic Stress in Those Who Treat the Traumatized*, ed. Charles R. Figley (New York: Brunner/Mazel, Inc., 1995), 51-81.

12. Karen L. Schuder, "Qualitative Study of Business Ethics Education: Preparing Leaders to Make Ethical Decisions" (EdD diss., University of St. Thomas, 2014).

13. Schuder, "Qualitative Study of Business Ethics Education."

14. Don R. Catherall, "Coping with Secondary Traumatic Stress: The Importance of the Therapist's Professional Peer Group," in *Secondary Traumatic Stress: Self-Care Issues for Clinicians, Researchers, and Educators*, 2nd ed., ed. B. Hudnall Stamm (Baltimore, MD: Sidran Press, 1999), 80-92.

15. Skovholt and Trotter-Mathison, *The Resilient Practitioner.*

16. Yassen, "Preventing Secondary Traumatic Stress."

17. Linda Graham, *Resilience: Powerful Practices for Bouncing Back from Disappointment, Difficulty, and Even Disaster* (Novato, CA: New World Library, 2018).

18. Jeffrey T. Mitchell, "Critical Incident Stress Debriefing (CISD)," *Info-Trauma.org*, accessed August 4, 2021, https://www.info-trauma.org

19. Susan L. McCammon and E. Jackson Allison, *"Debriefing and Treating Emergency Workers,"* in *Compassion Fatigue: Coping with Secondary Traumatic Stress in Those Who Treat the Traumatized*, ed. Charles R. Figley (New York: Brunner/Mazel, Inc., 1995), 115-130.

20. Catherall, "Coping with Secondary Traumatic Stress"; Beaton and Murphy, "Working with People in Crisis."

21. Mike Dubi, Patrick Powell, and J. Eric Gentry, *Trauma, PTSD, Grief & Loss: The 10 Core Competencies for Evidence-Based Treatment* (Eau Claire, WI: PESI Publishing & Media, 2017).

22. Catherall, "Coping with Secondary Traumatic Stress"; McCammon and Allison, "Debriefing and Treating Emergency Workers."

23. Graham, *Resilience*.

24. "The Twelve Steps," Al-Anon, accessed March 7, 2022, https://al-anon.org/for-members/the-legacies/the-twelve-steps/.

25. "Al-Anon History," Al-Anon, accessed August 10, 2021, https://al-anon.org/formembers/wso/ archives/history/.

26. Parker J. Palmer, *A Hidden Wholeness: The Journey Toward an Undivided Life* (San Francisco, CA: Jossey-Bass, 2004), 55.

27. Palmer, *A Hidden Wholeness.*

28. Van Dernoot Lipsky and Burk, *Trauma Stewardship.*

29. Graham, *Resilience.*

30. Palmer, *A Hidden Wholeness.*

31. Michael E. Kerr & Murray Bowen, *Family Evaluation: The Role of the Family as an Emotional Unit that Governs Individual Behavior and Development* (New York: W.W. Norton & Company, 1988).

32. Hanson, *Resilient.*

33. Palmer, *A Hidden Wholeness.*

ABOUT THE AUTHOR

Karen Schuder, EdD, MDiv, MAM

Karen's journey of helping people and her quest for sustainable caring started at a young age. Her experiences working with severely, multiply handicapped children, providing grief support to families after trauma, helping women recover from abuse, and dealing with collective grief have inspired her to build resilience and care sustainably. Her ultimate motivation is trying to find a way to enjoy her own life journey and wonderful family while walking with others in their suffering and brokenness.

Karen's drive to thrive while caring and her love for learning led to several graduate degrees, along with specialized training in multiple areas. She has an educational doctorate in leadership with research on ethics and professional development. Master's degrees in divinity and management expanded her educational perspective and skill set.

Karen has extensive experience helping people deal with trauma, coaching others to function at their best, and leading organizations. She has developed and led a wellness program for a family-physician residency program, provides ongoing leadership training in Honduras, and leads resilience workshops in educational settings and private practices.

Karen's areas of specialized training and experience include countering compassion fatigue, providing post-trauma and grief support, increasing cultural competency, handling conflict, shaping organizational cultures, and applying Family Systems Theory to leadership.

"I am focused on supporting people who help others, because I know how rewarding and challenging this can be," explains Karen. Years of dedicated searching for a way to thrive while helping people have led to *Resilient and Sustainable Caring*. She hopes to help others experience the beauty of their own lives—even when they walk amid suffering—and change the world with care.

Karen enjoys taking time to energize and spending time in nature with family, friends, and furry loved ones, going on hikes, skiing, and canoeing. We are surrounded by so much beauty!

Thank you for purchasing
Resilient and Sustainable Caring:
Your Guide to Thrive While Helping Others.

A portion of your purchase will go toward sending copies of this book to assist people in helping roles in Central America and other parts of the world where the need is great, but resources are not as easily available.

CPSIA information can be obtained
at www.ICGtesting.com
Printed in the USA
BVHW030314191022
649625BV00003B/9